# Understanding Asthma

Understanding Health and Sickness Series
*Miriam Bloom, Ph.D.*
*General Editor*

# Understanding Asthma

**Phil Lieberman, M.D.**

University Press of Mississippi
Jackson

http://www.upress.state.ms.us

Copyright © 1999 by the University Press of Mississippi
All rights reserved
Manufactured in the United States of America
02  01  00  99    4  3  2  1
The paper in this book meets the guidelines for permanence and durability
of the Committee on Production Guidelines for Book Longevity of the
Council on Library Resources.

Illustrations by Regan Causey Tuder.

Library of Congress Cataloging-in-Publication Data

Lieberman, Phil
    Understanding asthma / Phil Lieberman.
       p.   cm.—(Understanding health and sickness series)
    ISBN 1-57806-141-5 (cloth : alk. paper).—ISBN 1-57806-142-3
(pbk. : alk. paper)
    1. Asthma—Popular works.  I. Title.  II. Series.
RC591.L54  1999
616.2'38—dc21                     99-13753
                                      CIP

British Library Cataloging-in-Publication Data available

# Contents

# Introduction

Asthma is on the rise. The prevalence of asthma in children and young adults has increased dramatically over the past 20 to 30 years. Hospital admissions and deaths, especially of children, have risen everywhere, and today asthma exerts a huge impact on the health not only of Americans but of individuals around the world. It is estimated that as many as 21.5 million Americans suffer from this disease. Thirty-five percent of these are younger than 21 years of age; asthma has become the number one chronic illness of children and the number three chronic disease in the general population. It accounts for approximately 15 million physician office visits, almost 500,000 hospitalizations, almost 1.3 million emergency room visits, and over 10 million missed school days annually. More than 5,000 Americans died in 1997 from asthma attacks.

The prevalence of asthma is greater in women (5.6 percent) than in men (5.1 percent) and in blacks (5.8 percent) than in whites (5.1 percent). Blacks also have significantly more emergency room visits, hospitalizations, and deaths from asthma than do whites. From 1993 to 1995, an average of 38.5 deaths per million from asthma occurred in blacks compared to 15.1 per million in whites. In 1995, blacks were over 4 times more likely than whites to visit an emergency room because of asthma.

The economic cost of this condition is staggering. The direct cost, which includes hospital care, physician services, and medications to treat asthma, is about $5.2 billion per year. Indirect costs, such as those related to lost work and school days, approximate $0.7 billion per year. All of this has happened in spite of significant advances in our understanding of the illness and improvements in its therapy.

This paradox—the illness expanding in spite of improvements in therapy—prompted the National Institutes of Health in 1991 to mount the first nationwide coordinated attack on asthma. The outcome was the publication of *Guidelines for the Diagnosis and Management of Asthma*, a manuscript resulting from the deliberations of a blue-ribbon panel of physicians whose intent was to blunt the rising morbidity and mortality associated with this illness. Since that time, there have been no fewer than six such publications, including an international consensus, a global report, and a recently updated (1997) edition of the original guidelines. Each has emphasized the essential role of patient education. *Understanding Asthma* was conceived in the same spirit. I believe that only through understanding this disease will sufferers be able to control it. This book is intended for those who have the condition, for their families, and for any others who may have an interest in the subject.

The book explains the mechanisms of production of the condition and what happens in the lung, while also providing the rationale for therapy and self-management techniques based upon a knowledge of these mechanisms. I believe that unless the sufferer understands the process going on within the body and the underlying reasons for therapy, simple "how to" techniques will have little meaning and will soon be neglected. On the other hand, a knowledge of "why" imparts a real incentive to learn "how." I am in agreement with Dr. Albert L. Sheffer, chair of the first expert panel on the management of asthma, who states that "with appropriate therapy, patients with asthma can expect to control their symptoms, prevent most acute asthma exacerbations, manage the activity levels they desire, and attain near normal lung functioning." One of the major means of accomplishing this is through "patient education that fosters a partnership among the patient, family, and clinician."

Understanding involves knowing not only what to do but why we are doing it. The present work was undertaken with the goal of imparting knowledge about the inner workings of the disease.

I begin with a definition of the condition. The completion of this seemingly simple task has eluded organized medicine to date. In chapter 1, I share with the reader the evolution of the definition over time and analyze the present-day consensus definition.

Chapter 2, an exposition of the process occurring in the lung of the asthmatic, describes the pathology, pathophysiology, and cells and mediators involved in the production of the illness. Chapters 3 and 4 explore the precipitants of asthma episodes, with particular attention paid to the role of allergy, not only because it is one of the most important triggers but also because the allergic reaction in the lung serves as a model upon which the rationale of therapy is based. Chapter 5 contains a discussion of state-of-the-art measures used to control the illness. I emphasize the mechanisms of action of the various treatments, noting the differences between therapies that simply treat symptoms and those that may actually modify the disease. I discuss in detail the reasons for the differences between the actions of these two forms of therapy with the intention of imparting an understanding of *why* asthma should be treated in certain ways rather than simply *how* it is presently treated. Chapter 6 provides information about the tools that asthma sufferers and physicians use in diagnosis, monitoring, and therapy. The final chapter is an attempt at prophecy—a look into the future of treatments now being developed. Finally, the appendix lists organizations that are specifically dedicated to assisting asthmatics with the "how to" of management.

My major resource for this text is the experience of 30 years of studying the disease, living with it as a patient, raising an asthmatic child, and caring for thousands of sufferers. I also consulted many sources, drawing extensively on the aforementioned guidelines published by the National Institutes of Health (National Heart, Lung, and Blood Institute), including both editions of the expert panel report entitled *Guidelines for the Diagnosis and Management of Asthma* (the latest published in April 1997), the *International Consensus Report on Diagnosis and Management of Asthma* (March 1992), and the *Global Initiative for Asthma* (January 1995). Other informative sources were various symposia published by the *Journal of Allergy, Asthma and Immunology*, the *Annals of Asthma, Allergy and*

*Immunology,* and the *American Journal of Respiratory and Critical Care Medicine.* Of great help have been the thousands of sufferers who have so graciously allowed me to observe the capricious ebbs and flows of their condition so that I might learn from them while attempting to make things a little better.

# Understanding Asthma

# Defining Asthma

*If from running, gymnastic exercises, or any other work,
the breathing becomes difficult, it is called* Asthma; . . .
*for the paroxysms the patients also pant for breath . . . the
symptoms of its approach are heaviness of the chest . . .
difficulty breathing in running or on a steep road . . . and
troubled with cough.*

The Extant Works of Aretaeus,
the Cappadocian, circa 200 C.E.

We find references to asthma as early as the time of Hippocrates
(460–370 B.C.E.). The word itself is of Greek derivation and
refers to the act of "panting." Although we know that asthma
results from a narrowing of the opening of the airways due
to swelling, muscle contraction, and mucus in the bronchial
tubes, a definitive definition remains elusive. In the modern era,
organized medicine has made several valiant attempts dating
back to 1958 to establish a consensus definition. The last of these,
published in 1997 as part of the National Institutes of Health
Expert Panel Report, was entitled *Guidelines for the Diagnosis
and Management of Asthma.* Even with the intense effort of that
blue ribbon panel, the best that could be constructed was a
working definition. The reason for the difficulty is that asthma
is not, in the commonly recognized sense, a specific disease;
that is, it differs significantly from illnesses such as tuberculosis
which have a single cause. Rather, it is a "condition," an
incompletely understood abnormality, and its exact cause is
unknown. In fact, there are probably multiple causes. Thus our

definitions cannot address the genesis of the illness, and are limited to descriptions of its characteristics and manifestations. However, the situation is not as bleak as it might appear, for these descriptive definitions are becoming increasingly more perceptive as our knowledge expands regarding the mechanisms of production of the condition.

I think it is important for readers to know the evolution of our definitions and therefore our understanding of this illness. Perhaps the most salient premodern definition was offered by Sir William Osler in the late 1800s when he defined asthma as a "special form of *inflammation* of the small bronchioles" and called it "bronchiolitis exudativa." The use of the term "inflammation" was somewhat prescient; only recently have we learned the importance of the inflammatory aspects of the illness. In fact, for the many decades between Osler's definition and the 1980s, the inflammatory nature of asthma was forgotten, and the condition was considered to be an inherent abnormality of the smooth muscle surrounding the bronchi (a concept which will be discussed in more detail later).

The first modern attempt to arrive at a consensus definition of asthma occurred in 1958 at a guest symposium organized by the CIBA Foundation: "Asthma refers to the condition of subjects with *widespread narrowing* of the *bronchial airways*, which changes in severity over short periods of time either spontaneously or under treatment, and is not due to cardiovascular disease. The clinical characteristics are abnormal breathlessness, which may be paroxysmal or persistent, wheezing, and in most cases relief by bronchodilator drugs (including corticosteroids)." The absence of any mention of inflammation reflects medicine's temporary amnesia regarding Osler's early observations.

In 1962, the Committee on Diagnostic Standards of the American Thoracic Society produced the following definition: "Asthma is a disease characterized by an *increased responsiveness* of the trachea and *bronchi* to various stimuli and manifested by *widespread narrowing* of the airways that changes in severity either spontaneously or as a result of therapy." This definition was considered by another convening of the CIBA Foundation study group in 1971 and was rejected by some participants. They did not feel that asthma could be accepted as a "disease" for the reasons previously mentioned.

In 1986, the American Thoracic Society again attempted to define the condition, and in the new definition noted for the first time the infiltration of the lung by *"inflammatory cells."*

Then, in 1991, the first blue ribbon committee was impaneled by the National Institutes of Health to define the condition and establish guidelines for its diagnosis and management. Emerging from the conference was this statement: "Asthma is a lung disease with the following characteristics: (1) airway *obstruction* that is *reversible* (but not completely so in some patients) either spontaneously or with treatment; (2) airway *inflammation*; and (3) *increased airway responsiveness* to a variety of stimuli."

Finally, in 1997, the committee was reconvened and charged with revising the guidelines and the definition, which remains the most current consensus:

> Asthma is a chronic *inflammatory disorder* of the airways in which *many cells* and cellular elements play a role, in particular, mast cells, eosinophils, T-lymphocytes, macrophages, neutrophils, and epithelial cells. In susceptible individuals, this inflammation causes recurrent episodes of *wheezing, breathlessness, chest tightness*, and *coughing*, particularly at night or in the early morning. These episodes are usually associated with *widespread but variable air flow obstruction* that is often *reversible* either spontaneously or with treatment. The *inflammation* also causes an associated increase in the existing *bronchial hyperresponsiveness* to a variety of stimuli. Moreover, recent evidence indicates that sub-basement membrane *fibrosis* may occur in some patients with asthma and that these changes contribute to persistent abnormalities in lung function.

Features of this definition that distinguish it from previous attempts are the emphasis on the inflammatory component of the illness and the mention of particular cells as agents in the production of the illness. In addition, for the first time, a reference is made to the fact that asthma may cause permanent lung damage in the form of fibrosis (scarring). Finally, the definition reemphasizes the term "bronchial hyperresponsiveness," which is a hallmark of the illness.

Let us examine these terms so that we may formulate a concept of the illness based on a description of its hallmarks as included in the definition. All asthmatics share certain characteristics that are fundamental to the disease process. These are as follows:

**Table 1.1** The Hallmarks of Asthma

---

Inflammation

Airway obstruction

Bronchial hyperresponsiveness

Potential for fibrosis

---

1. *Inflammation.* Inflammation is characterized by swelling and weeping. It can be a protective response caused by the influx of cells to an area of the body. However, under certain circumstances, asthma being one of them, the inflammatory response is damaging. The symptoms produced by inflammation depend upon where it occurs. For example, in the skin, inflammation would produce redness, weeping (an exudate), pain, a burning sensation, and/or itch. In the lung, inflammation narrows the tubes (bronchi) that carry inhaled air deep into the lungs, causing shortness of breath, wheezing, and cough. The invading cells, as noted in the most recent definition of asthma, include mast cells, eosinophils, T-lymphocytes, macrophages, neutrophils, and epithelial cells. We now know that these cells are major players in the production of the condition. In essence, one might view the lung itself as being a "good neighbor" in a "bad neighborhood," the bad neighbors being the cells that have, although unwelcomed, moved into the neighborhood of

the lung. Key to our understanding of the disease will be the role of each cell in the production of the problem, to be discussed later. All asthmatics express this inflammatory component.

2. *Airway obstruction (narrowing of the bronchi)*. All of the most recent definitions of this illness mention the widespread narrowing of the bronchi that leads to variable air flow obstruction. How such narrowing is produced will be discussed in detail. It is important to note, however, that the narrowing can occur suddenly, is reversible in most cases, and causes wheezing, shortness of breath, tightness in the chest, and cough. The narrowing is provoked by diverse stimuli, to which "twitchy" asthmatic lungs are hyperresponsive.

3. *Bronchial hyperresponsiveness*. This term refers to the peculiar predisposition of asthmatics to respond to diverse stimuli with constriction of the muscles surrounding the bronchial tubes and later with increased secretion and the influx of the aforementioned cells. The stimuli can include weather conditions, strong odors and fumes, exercise, upper respiratory tract infections (the common cold), and, in some patients, *allergy*—an exaggerated immunologic response to normally harmless substances such as pollen, animal danders, dust mites, and mold spores.

4. *Fibrosis (scarring)*. Although in most instances episodes of narrowing are reversible, in some patients scarring and permanent lung damage from tissue destruction can occur over a long period of time. This aspect of the illness was first noted in the 1991 definition and was emphasized in the 1997 definition. The nature of this scarring and its prevention has become an important issue over the last few years and has prompted a different philosophy (discussed later) regarding therapy.

Although these four characteristics are shared by all asthmatics, it is still important to recognize that asthma is not a homogeneous entity. It exists in many forms. As noted, some asthmatics have allergies, whereas others do not. In many, the condition is extremely mild and does not significantly interfere with quality of life. In other cases, the illness can be debilitating.

It is because of this heterogeneity that a true definition of the illness remains unattainable at our present level of knowledge. Nonetheless, we clearly understand the characteristics of the condition and many of its causes, and we can describe it extremely well. Thus we have come a long way since Aretaeus.

Let us now take a detailed look at the processes that occur in the asthmatic lung.

# What Happens in the Lung?

*An Asthma is a most terrible disease . . . for there is scarce anything more sharp and terrible than the fits hereof . . . But as to evident causes they are many, and also of diverse sorts . . . Asthmatical persons can endure nothing violent or unaccustomed: From excesses of cold, or heat, from any vehement motion of body or mind, by any great change of Air, or of the year, or from the slightest errors about the things not natural, yea from a thousand other occasions they fall into fits of difficult breathing . . . Whatsoever therefore makes the blood to boyl, or raises it into an effervescence, as violent motion of the body or mind, excess of extern cold or heat, the drinking of Wine, Venery, yea sometimes mere heat of the Bed doth cause asthmatical assaults to such as are predisposed.*

Thomas Willis, English physician, 1684

To understand how asthma affects the lung, it is necessary to know what that organ does. The lung can be viewed as a passive bellows designed for two purposes: (1) it serves as a passageway through which air can flow from the external environment into the body, and (2) it serves as a transfer station for oxygen (that we breathe in) and carbon dioxide (that we breathe out).

To visualize the anatomy of the lung, think of an upside-down tree. The trunk is the *trachea*, which then divides into branches, or *bronchioles*. At the end of the bronchioles are the air sacs, or *alveoli* (fig. 2.1). Air passes from the widest point at the trachea into gradually narrowing bronchioles until it reaches the air sacs. As air fills these sacs, they expand and their walls thin, much like what happens when air is blown into a balloon. As the walls of the alveoli stretch and become thinner, they allow diffusion of oxygen into the bloodstream while carbon dioxide diffuses from the bloodstream into the air sac. Thus on inhalation we refresh the bloodstream with oxygen, and upon exhalation we remove carbon dioxide produced by the body's metabolism, releasing it into the air.

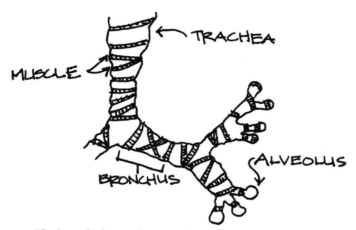

FIG. 2.1. The bronchial tree, showing the trachea and its division into smaller tubes (bronchi and bronchioles), which terminate in air sacs (alveoli). Muscle capable of contracting and thus of squeezing the bronchus surrounds the tubes.

Asthma is a condition involving the branches (bronchioles) of the bronchial tree. In asthma, these bronchioles become narrowed for many reasons, which I will discuss below. For the sake of simplicity, let's assume that we are looking at the tree as one tube in comparing an asthmatic airway with a normal airway (fig. 2.2). In asthma the narrowing of the tube makes breathing more difficult. What is known as our "work of breathing," or the energy and effort that must be put into each breath, increases, and the sufferer experiences shortness of breath, one of the cardinal symptoms of this condition. In addition, air traversing the narrowed bronchial tubes can produce a high-pitched sound known as a wheeze, one of the seminal findings physicians look for when they listen to the chest. The bronchial tubes are wider open when we breathe in than when we breathe out; thus the narrowing that occurs in asthma is accentuated when the breath is expelled. This leads to the trapping of air in the lung, which leaves some of the air sacs filled with air and makes patients feel as if they are "breathing off the top of their lungs." No matter how hard they attempt to breathe, the already-filled air sacs cannot be expanded further because of trapped air.

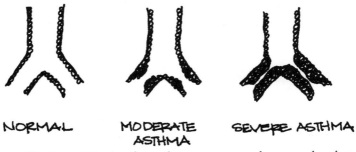

NORMAL     MODERATE ASTHMA     SEVERE ASTHMA

FIG. 2.2. The bronchial tube of an asthmatic is narrowed compared to that of a nonasthmatic. The more prominent the narrowing is, the more severe the asthma will be.

## What Causes the Narrowing?

Now that we know that asthma is a condition characterized by narrowing of the bronchial tubes which causes wheezing, shortness of breath, and coughing, let's look at what produces this narrowing. Actually, it is the result of a combination of factors: constriction of the circular muscles surrounding the tube, thickening of the tube's wall, excess production of mucus, swelling (*edema*) of the tube's lining, and scarring (*fibrosis*) of the tubes. Figure 2.3 shows a cross section of a normal bronchial tube compared with an asthmatic tube.

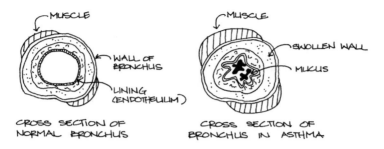

FIG. 2.3. Cross sections of the normal bronchus and the asthmatic bronchus, demonstrating the factors that produce narrowing of the bronchial tubes in asthma. These include muscle thickening and contraction, thickening of the bronchus wall, excess production of mucus, and swelling of the tube's lining.

### Constriction of the circular muscles surrounding the bronchial tube

The normal bronchial tube is surrounded by muscle. When the muscle contracts, it narrows the diameter of the tube. As with all muscle, continued contraction will cause growth, or *hypertrophy*. The muscle itself becomes chronically thickened, even in its resting state, which narrows the tube further.

Contraction of the muscles surrounding the bronchial tube can occur with amazing rapidity. When a stimulus is encountered, within a few seconds profound narrowing of the tubes due to muscle constriction can occur. Such narrowing, in its most severe form, can result in a person's sudden death from asphyxiation. This rapid response to stimuli that fail to produce such a reaction in the nonasthmatic is known as *bronchial hyperresponsiveness*, which is, as noted in chapter 1, a hallmark of the disease and a feature shared by all asthmatics. That is, exposure to normally innocuous agents can, in the asthmatic, rapidly produce threatening impairment of breathing through constriction of the muscles surrounding the bronchi. Heterogeneous stimuli that are capable of causing this type of sudden adverse event include changes in temperature and humidity, exposure to irritating fumes or odors, the common cold, and exercise. This characteristic has been used to diagnose asthma because it helps us separate patients who experience shortness of breath, coughing, or wheezing for reasons other than asthma from those who are asthmatic. The hyperresponsiveness can be measured in the laboratory by graded exposure of patients to agents known to precipitate a hyperresponsive event with contraction of the smooth muscle surrounding the bronchial tubes. Like all muscle in the body, it has the power to contract. When it does so, the bronchial tubes are "choked" as their lumen narrows. The chemicals most commonly used to perform this diagnostic test are *histamine* and *methacholine*. When an asthmatic inhales these substances, contraction of the muscles occurs within seconds, a reaction that does not normally occur in a nonasthmatic. The test itself therefore has been useful in establishing a diagnosis by distinguishing shortness of breath due to other causes from that due to asthma.

### Thickening of the bronchial tube wall

In asthma, the walls of the breathing tubes become swollen for a number of reasons. First of all, cells from outside the lung enter the bronchial tubes and take up residence there, expanding the diameter of the tube. Some of these cells, in addition, manufacture chemicals commonly referred to as *ground substances*, which have a function similar to that of mortar and cement in the construction of a building—they hold the elements of the lung together. In asthma the cells produce an excessive amount of these chemicals, thus widening the wall of the bronchi further.

*Excess mucus production*

Mucus facilitates transport of substances along the inner surface of the bronchi and lubricates the surface. In asthma, not only is excess mucus produced, but its thickness makes it tenacious and difficult to cough up. The mucus fills the tube, narrowing the airway further.

*Swelling (edema) of the tube's lining*

Edema is swelling due to accumulation of fluid. In asthma, fluid accumulates under and in the lining of the bronchial tube. Some of the fluid is produced by cells that infiltrate the lining of the lung, and some comes through leakage of serum from the blood vessels in the area. This excess accumulation of fluid is part of the inflammatory response, and is analogous to the weeping from a wound in the skin.

In many asthma attacks these changes occur sequentially. Usually, the first thing to occur during an asthma attack is the rapid contraction of the muscles surrounding the bronchial tubes, followed shortly by excess secretion and accumulation of edema fluid. Usually the easiest of these abnormalities to correct and the first to subside is the contraction of the muscles. The excess mucus and edema disappear more slowly.

*Scarring (fibrosis) and tissue destruction*

As we have seen, one of the newer observations noted in the most recent consensus definition of asthma is the fact that this illness can produce permanent structural changes in the bronchial tubes. These changes occur over time. They seem to be caused by at least two processes. One is a scarring associated with overproduction of the ground substances noted above. This scarring occurs as a result of multiple episodes of asthma with damage, followed by healing. At times the healing is incomplete and permanent scars form, producing shrinkage of the lung. In addition, some of the chemicals that are secreted during the asthmatic episode can damage the lung's *elastic tissue*, which provides a counterbalancing force that opposes constriction of the muscles. Elastic tissue is much like a coiled spring: the thicker the diameter of the spring, the more difficult stretching it is. These elastic springs tether the peripheral portion of the bronchial lumen to the tissue of the lung and thus act to hold the bronchi open.

This excess laying down of ground substance with scarring accompanied by destruction of the elastic tissue can produce permanent changes which, over time, cause irreversible impairment of breathing. Whether or not this can be prevented with therapy or reversed is an issue of intense debate and a subject for future research. However, scarring and destruction do not occur in all individuals with asthma.

## The Cells that Cause Asthma

As noted, one of the present ways of thinking about asthma is to see the lung as an "innocent bystander" harmed by cells that "attack" it. The aggressor cells (table 2.1) are lymphocytes, eosinophils, mast cells, epithelial cells, fibroblasts, macrophages, and neutrophils. A brief description of each cell and the role it plays in the production of asthma will help us understand this illness.

Lymphocytes are the cells that control the immune response. They are divided into two populations: T-lymphocytes and B-lymphocytes. B-lymphocytes manufacture antibodies that help protect us from certain illnesses. One of these antibodies, as we shall see later, is the allergic antibody (IgE) that causes allergies.T-lymphocytes are, for lack of a better term, the conductor of the immune orchestra. They send signals to all other cells causing them to behave in a helpful or a harmful way. For example, T-lymphocytes send messages to B-lymphocytes telling them how much antibody to make, thus being ultimately responsible in large part for the amount of allergic antibody

**Table 2.1** Cells that Produce Inflammation in Asthma

| Cell | Activity |
| --- | --- |
| Lymphocyte | Orchestrates the aberrant immune response |
| Eosinophil | The major effector cell, containing chemicals that produce the reaction; their number in the lung correlates with the activity of the illness |
| Mast cell | Releases chemicals, such as histamine, which contract bronchial smooth muscle and call forth other cells |
| Epithelial cell | Lines the inner surface of the lung and secretes chemicals that activate other cells |
| Fibroblast | Produces ground substances and thus can cause scarring |
| Macrophage | Scavenger cell producing chemicals that amplify the inflammation |
| Neutrophil | May be active in some cases of severe, acute episodes |

manufactured by B-lymphocytes. The T-lymphocyte population is divided into two subcategories of cells: *suppressor/cytotoxic T-cells* and *helper T-cells*. Suppressor cytotoxic T-cells dampen the immune response and play a role in the destruction of other cells which have become ill, such as, for example, cells infected with viruses. Helper T-cells, on the other hand, enhance the immune response. Normally the helper T-cell initiates a beneficial response designed to control infections.

There are two classes of helper T-cells, TH1 and TH2. TH1 cells are instrumental in our defense against what are known as intracellular infections, which are produced by microorganisms such as the tuberculosis bacterium that invade and live within our cells. TH2 cells are normally employed in the defense against other organisms, specifically parasites more commonly associated with tropical infections. These include agents such as the worms that cause trichinosis, which we can get from eating uncooked pork. As we will see later, an aberrant TH2 cell response can also cause allergic asthma. This aberrant response results in the overproduction of the allergic antibody.

These cells (fig. 2.4) produce *cytokines*, chemicals that have a profound effect on the body's immune response (table 2.2). The major chemicals produced by TH1 cells are interleukin-2 (IL-2) and gamma interferon. These two cytokines are necessary for the defense against infection with intracellular organisms. On the other hand, TH2 cells produce IL-4, IL-5, IL-10 and IL-13. These cytokines, which help kill parasites, are associated with respiratory allergies. In other words, an overabundance or hyperactivity of the TH2 cell population induces an aberrant immune response capable of producing allergic disease. The cytokines that are manufactured by TH2 cells cause an increase in the production of allergic antibody, *IgE*, and mobilize and activate the major effector cell (the eosinophil) responsible for asthma. Allergic asthmatics have an imbalance in their T-cell profile, favoring the TH2 cell.

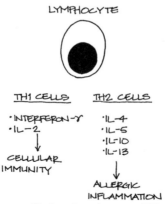

FIG. 2.4. The two types of helper lymphocytes. TH1 cells manufacture substances such as interferon and IL-2, which aid in the defense against certain infections. TH2 cells, presumably evolved as a defense against parasites, manufacture IL-4, IL-5, IL-10, and IL-13. These interleukins produce elements of the allergic response (see table 2.2).

**Table 2.2** Cells that Produce Inflammation in Asthma

| Cytokine* | Cell-Producing | Biologic Activity |
|---|---|---|
| Interferon | TH1 | Aids in destruction of viruses and other organisms (such as the tuberculosis bacterium) that infect cells |
| IL-2 | TH1 | Activates other lymphocytes to assist in the destruction of intracellular organisms as with interferon |
| IL-4 | TH2 | Enhances the production of the allergic antibody (IgE)** |
| IL-5 | TH2 | Activates eosinophils and prolongs their survival |
| IL-10 | TH2 | Reduces the production of interferon by TH2 lymphocytes |
| IL-13 | TH2 | Mimics the activity of IL-4 |

*IL stands for interleukin
**The allergic antibody is discussed in chapter 3

It is important to note that not all asthmatics have allergies; those who don't are commonly referred to as *intrinsic asthmatics*. (This subject will be discussed in more detail later.) Allergic asthmatics produce excess amounts of both IL-4, which enhances the production of allergic antibody, and IL-5, which enhances the activity of eosinophils. Nonallergic or intrinsic asthmatics only have overproduction of IL-5, with IL-4 levels being normal.

*Eosinophils* are normally used in our defense against parasites. They are also the major effector cells in the vast majority of asthma cases. That is, their entrance into the lung produces the damage. These cells contain toxic substances which, when released, cause damage to the bronchial tree. The number of eosinophils present within the bronchial secretions and bloodstream correlates well with disease severity.

*Mast cells* are involved in one of the primary steps in the production of asthma. We will learn more about the mast cell when we examine in detail the nature of the allergic response. At this point we need only say that mast cells contain chemicals which can cause numerous adverse effects in the lungs. When these chemicals, which include *histamine, leukotrienes, platelet activating factor, kallikreins,* and others, are released from the mast cells, they produce constriction of the smooth muscle surrounding the bronchi, leakage of serum from the vessels of the lungs into the bronchi, and recruitment of other cells such as lymphocytes and eosinophils to the lung. Mast cells live inside the lumen of the bronchi, and thus are quite readily exposed to inhaled substances that can initiate the asthmatic episode. Exposure to such substances in susceptible individuals causes the mast cells to release their contents, thus initiating a cascade of events, the result of which is coughing, wheezing, and shortness of breath.

*Epithelial cells* line the breathing tubes. They are capable of secreting many substances which then can activate other cells. One such substance is known to activate fibroblasts.

*Fibroblasts* reside in the lungs, skin, and other organs. One of their major roles is to manufacture support tissue such as ground substances to repair wounds. They are thus active in the healing process. However, if they become overactive and manufacture ground substances inappropriately, tissue scarring can occur. In asthmatics, fibroblasts are present in increased numbers and exhibit excessive activity in the bronchi.

*Macrophages* are scavenger cells that clean up debris and kill invaders, which they do by ingesting foreign substances and destroying them through digestion. In doing so they manufacture chemicals that in turn activate the inflammatory response. For example, like mast cells, macrophages can manufacture leukotrienes, which can constrict the smooth muscle surrounding the bronchi. There is evidence that macrophages are hyperactive in asthmatic patients.

*Neutrophils* are much like macrophages in that they capture, ingest, and kill substances which the body sees as foreign. They do not usually seem to play a role in asthma, but in certain asthmatics who experience sudden death, presumably due to severe, rapid constriction of the bronchial muscles, these cells are found in the lung in abundance.

Perhaps the best way to visualize this very complex cellular infiltration and the resultant inflammatory response is to think of the lung as a tissue which faces the external environment. With each inhalation we draw into our lungs whatever may be in the air at that time. The body must be very busy to purify each breath and to react should it detect an invader. The reaction consists of the lung calling forth these cells to deal with invaders. However, in the process of doing their job, the cells can also produce disease. The contents of these cells are not selective—that is, they are toxic not only to an invader but also to the host.

In asthma, these cells are involved in exaggerated and inappropriate activity, and their invasion of the lung results in illness.

All of the aforementioned cells produce their inflammatory effects through the synthesis and release of chemicals known as *inflammatory mediators*: histamine, leukotrienes, platelet activating factor, major basic protein and cationic protein, prostaglandins, TGF-beta, elastase, and chemotactic factors. Knowledge of these chemicals and their activities is germane to our understanding of asthma (table 2.3).

*Histamine* was probably the first inflammatory mediator isolated from the mast cell. It causes a number of effects that produce manifestations of asthma, including contraction of smooth muscle, increased permeability of the blood vessels (which causes leakage of serum into the lung), irritation of the lung's nerve endings (which can cause coughing), and an increase in the production of mucus. Histamine is found solely in mast cells and basophils (cells that are probably active in the

**Table 2.3** Chemical Mediators of Asthma and Their Biologic Effects

| Mediator | Cell that produces it | Effect |
| --- | --- | --- |
| Histamine | Mast cell | Contraction of muscles surrounding bronchi |
| | | Leakage of serum from blood vessels |
| | | Mucus secretion |
| | | Irritation of nerves causing cough |
| Leukotrienes | Mast cell Eosinophil | Similar to histamine but causes more profound and prolonged muscle contraction |
| | Macrophage | Increase in bronchial hyperresponsiveness |
| Platelet activating factor | Mast cell Eosinophil | Muscle contraction |
| | | Increase in bronchial hyperresponsiveness |
| | | Leakage of serum |
| Major basic protein Cationic protein | Eosinophil | Damage to tissue, especially epithelial cells, of the bronchioles |
| Prostaglandins | Mast cell Eosinophil | Muscle contraction |
| | | Leakage of serum |
| Transforming growth factor-beta | Bronchial lining cells Mast cell | Stimulation of fibroblasts to manufacture collagen (a ground substance) |
| Elastase | Neutrophils and other cells | Destruction of elastic tissue |
| Chemotactic factors | Mast cell | Attracting of cells (eosinophils, fibroblasts, etc.) to bronchi |

production of allergic reactions in the nose but probably not in the production of asthma).

*Leukotrienes* cause effects similar to those caused by histamine; in addition, they also call eosinophils to the site of the reaction and increase bronchial hyperresponsiveness. One of the most recent advances in asthma therapy is the development of antileukotriene drugs (see chapter 5). Leukotrienes are manufactured mainly in mast cells, eosinophils, and macrophages.

*Platelet activating factor* can increase the permeability of blood vessels (causing the formation of edema), cause smooth muscle to contract, and increase bronchial hyperresponsiveness.

Eosinophils contain *major basic protein* and *cationic protein*, which are highly toxic to the lining of the bronchial tubes. During bouts of asthma, eosinophils release these substances into the tissues. The damage they cause plays a key role in the production of the illness.

A definite role for *prostaglandins* in the production of asthma has not been established. However, they can cause a number of different effects that at least theoretically could contribute to the disease; these include constriction of smooth muscle as well as increased permeability of the blood vessels.

*Transforming growth factor-beta (TGF-beta)* is made by a number of different cells including the cells lining the bronchial tree. TGF-beta can activate fibroblasts and cause them to produce and release the ground substances discussed above; as we have seen, this can cause chronic, irreversible changes in the lung.

*Elastase*, made by neutrophils and other cells, has been found in the bronchial secretions of asthmatics during acute episodes. Elastase breaks down the elastic tissue that opposes the contraction of smooth muscle.

Mast cells release substances that are called *chemotactic factors* because they are chemicals (*chemo*) that cause cells to move (*taxi*). In asthma, they move cells from the bloodstream into the lung. A number of different chemotactic factors have been found in the bronchial secretions of asthmatics. Most of these agents are especially chemotactic for eosinophils and include substances known as *chemokines* and other elements named for their activity (eosinophil—chemotactic factors). The chemotactic factors are to these cells what the scent of blood is to a shark; the cells move toward the highest concentration of the chemicals.

In summary, in this chapter we have looked at the pathologic events that occur in asthma, the final result of which is a narrowing of the bronchial tubes producing coughing, wheezing, and shortness of breath. We have seen that the narrowing occurs due to several factors, including contraction of the muscle, swelling of the walls and lining of the tubes, and overproduction of mucus.

We have learned that it is the influx of cells and their production of chemical mediators that directly cause the pathology. The major effects of these mediators are contraction of smooth muscle, increased permeability of the blood vessels with resulting edema, production of bronchial hyperresponsiveness, and laying down of ground substances with subsequent scarring.

We have seen that in asthmatics the conductor of the immune response, the lymphocyte, often differs from that found in nonasthmatics. In asthmatics the predominant lymphocyte is often of the TH2 subset, which produces chemicals that are associated with the allergic reaction rather than with the immune defense against intracellular organisms. This brings us to the next important step in our understanding of asthma: learning about allergy.

# Allergy and Its Relationship to Asthma

*An asthmatic is an individual who is sensitized to a definite substance and an asthmatic attack sets in every time this substance manages in some way to enter into the circulation of the individual.*

S. J. Meltzer, M.D., *The Journal of American Medical Association*, 1910

In the above quotation, Dr. Meltzer was describing what we now know to be the allergic asthmatic. The originator of the term "allergy" was the Austrian pediatrician Clemens von Pirqet. In 1907, he wrote "*Klinische Studien über Vakzination und vakzinale Allergie,*" thereby coining the term. The word derives from the Greek *allos,* meaning "other" or "altered," and *ergos,* meaning "work" or "activity." Von Pirqet put the two terms together to imply that "allergy" was an altered activity or reactivity. He originally intended that the word be used to encompass all altered reactivity of the body; for example, immunity due to a vaccination would be an allergic reaction (altered immunologic activity). Later, in the 1920s, two American physicians, A. F. Coca and R. A. Cooke (who was himself an asthmatic), refined the term and used it to refer to a group of illnesses characterized by an *abnormal reactivity* to *normally harmless substances.* They coined another term—atopy—to refer to a group of inherited diseases that were characterized by this type of altered reactivity. These later became known as the allergic diseases and today include allergic rhinitis, atopic dermatitis, and the disease in question, asthma.

The term "allergy" refers to an altered reactivity that is produced by a specific immune reaction. The substances producing an allergic response are termed *allergens*. These substances share two very important characteristics. They are almost always *organic* (alive or once alive) and are *always harmless to the nonallergic individual*. Examples of allergens known to produce asthma include the pollens of trees, grasses, and weeds, mold spores, house dust mites, and animal danders. It is important to distinguish these from *irritants* such as strong odors and fumes (cigarette smoke, hair spray, paint fumes), and pollutants (sulphur dioxide, ozone). Irritants do not cause adverse events only in the allergic individual; present in large enough amounts, they can cause such reactions in all of us, allergic or not. On the other hand, an allergen, which would be totally undetectable to the nonallergic individual, can cause profound symptoms in the allergic patient. The difference between a nonallergic individual's response and an allergic individual's response to an allergen is qualitative and to an irritant is quantitative. That is, we will all react to an irritant if exposed to a sufficient quantity of it. For example, the nonasthmatic may cough and wheeze if exposed to a sufficient quantity of sulfur dioxide, an irritant gas. The asthmatic simply reacts to a much smaller amount. On the other hand, no matter how much pollen people without the condition encounter, they will not react. Understanding this concept is important, since the distinction has implications for therapy. One can alter the immune response to an allergen by measures such as allergy injections, but this cannot be done for an irritant, in which case where the only therapy (with the exception of medication) is avoidance. Thus the distinction between allergens and irritants has therapeutic significance.

Not all asthmatics are allergic, nor is all asthma caused by allergy. In some patients asthma is due almost entirely to allergies, whereas others have no allergies at all. However, allergies are clearly one of the most—perhaps *the* most—important provocateurs of this illness. For example, approximately 90 percent of children with asthma have a strong allergic component, and approximately 50 to 60 percent of adults have asthma that can be provoked at least to some extent by allergies.

Traditionally, those patients in whom allergies are responsible for a significant portion of their asthma are called "extrinsic" asthmatics and those in whom no allergy can be identified as "intrinsic" asthmatics. This division of asthmatics into allergic (extrinsic) and nonallergic (intrinsic) was first made in 1918 by Dr. Francis Rackemann, a Boston-educated physician who was a pioneer in the development of the study of allergic diseases as a distinct branch of medicine, and, although there have been many attempts through the years to improve upon this terminology, no suitable alternatives have appeared. The use of the terms grew out of the observation that the causes of allergic asthmatic reactions were usually easily identified (as substance in the external environment) by allergy skin testing and history (an individual wheezes immediately upon exposure to a cat or to freshly cut grass), whereas the precipitants of intrinsic asthma are more difficult to identify, and originally it was thought that they actually came from within rather than from without the individual—thus the term "intrinsic."

Other agents known to produce asthma episodes (discussed in detail in chapter 5) include any strong odor or fume, weather conditions (such as a front coming in), air pollutants, exercise, certain chemicals such as isocyanates (usually encountered only in occupational asthma), and the common cold. Of these, the last is the most important. In fact, the common cold and allergy probably account for well over 90 percent of hospital admissions due to asthma and a vast majority of the daily morbidity experienced by patients with this disease.

Even though allergies are not the sole cause of this illness, and in some patients play no role at all, the study of the allergic respiratory response is of signal importance in our understanding of asthma. The allergic reaction per se forms a scientific paradigm for the study of the disease, and many of the pathologic responses due to allergy have also been identified in the nonallergic asthmatic. For example, we use allergic asthmatic reactions to study the effect of drugs in treating the disease since allergic challenges are simple to perform and are reproducible. In addition, the biopsy findings in allergic and nonallergic asthma are similar, and many of the chemicals responsible for the illness are the same for both types. Thus a grasp of the mechanism involved in the production of the allergic response is required for the understanding of asthma.

## The Allergic Reaction

The allergic reaction has a sensitization phase and an effector phase. It requires three components: the allergen, the allergic antibody (IgE), and the mast cell (fig. 3.1).

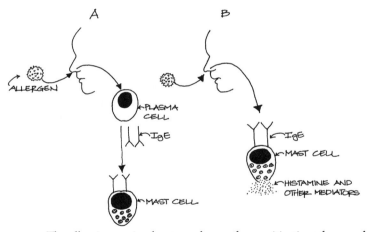

FIG. 3.1. The allergic reaction has two phases, the sensitization phase and the effector phase. In the sensitization phase (panel A), initial exposure to allergen initiates the production of allergic antibody (IgE) by the plasma cell of the immune system. The IgE travels through the bloodstream and attaches to mast cells lining the respiratory tract. With reexposure to allergen (panel B), the IgE attached to the mast cell binds to the allergen as well. This results in a process known as degranulation, whereby the cell releases its contents, which then produce the allergic reaction.

As we have seen, allergens are organic particles which are harmless to nonallergic individuals but which produce symptoms when inhaled by the allergic asthmatic. The most common ones were listed earlier in this chapter.

Antibodies ward off foreign invaders. They travel in the bloodstream or act as sentinels where our body faces the external environment (e.g., eyes, nose, throat) and combine with invaders, immobilizing them and enhancing the body's ability to destroy them. We produce antibodies against viruses, bacteria, and parasites. All antibodies are proteins and are called immunoglobulins. There are five classes, each designated by a letter: immunoglobulin G (IgG), immunoglobulin A (IgA), immunoglobulin M (IgM), immunoglobulin D (IgD), and immunoglobulin E (IgE). IgE protects us against multicellular parasites such as hookworms and trichinosis worms. For some reason unbeknownst to us, this same antibody, in a small portion of our population—those with allergies—is synthesized in response to simple allergens as well. Thus, allergy can be visualized as an aberrant immune response in which the antibody that normally fends off parasites is instead directed against harmless substances.

Antibodies are Y-shaped molecules. The arms of the Y combine with invaders such as viruses, bacteria, or parasites. The tail of the Y determines other features, including whether the antibody attaches to a cell. With IgE antibodies, the tail of the molecule affixes to cells such as eosinophils and mast cells (fig. 3.2). When the antibody attached to a mast cell or eosinophil encounters a parasite, it causes the cell to *degranulate*, a process whereby its chemicals are released. These chemicals then initiate a series of events that purge the invader from the body, poison it, or call forth other cells which in turn help destroy it. For example, histamine released from the mast cell purges parasites from the intestine by contracting smooth muscles surrounding the intestine, which in turn produces a progressive wave of narrowing of the intestine "squeezing" the parasite out (much like the squeezing of toothpaste from a tube). Histamine also causes the formation of excess mucus that "washes" the parasite from the bowel and increases blood flow to the site, resulting in increased permeability of the blood vessels. This allows other cells easier access to the site, and these can in turn attack the parasite. The major cell to do so is the eosinophil. The eosinophil also has a receptor for IgE antibody on its surface. Again, the tail end of the IgE antibody affixes to the eosinophil and the arms of the Y to the parasite. This union in turn causes the eosinophil to release its contents, one being major basic protein, which, as previously noted, is highly toxic and destroys the parasite.

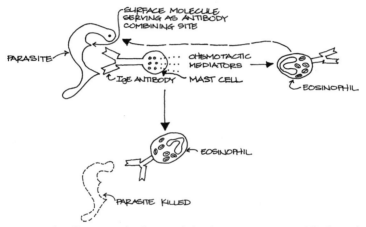

FIG. 3.2. The allergic antibody, IgE, defends against parasites. The branched end attaches to the parasite and the tail end to a cell that kills the parasite or purges it from the body. Two such cells are the eosinophil and the mast cell. When IgE on a mast cell encounters a parasite, the cell releases chemicals that destroy the parasite or purge it from the body. One of the effects is to call forth eosinophils, which then attack and destroy the parasite via the IgE affixed to the eosinophil surface.

In this scenario, the IgE-mast cell unit is beneficial to our survival. It is the prime defense mechanism against a certain class of invaders. However, this same series of events directed against an allergen results in an inappropriate activation of the inflammatory cascade and produces what we have previously mentioned as the allergic diseases. In allergic disease, the series of events begins in a similar fashion—that is, IgE, affixed to a mast cell surface, unites with allergen (rather than parasite), thus causing degranulation of the mast cell with release of the chemicals noted earlier, including histamine, leukotrienes, and others. These in turn produce an immediate response, with contraction of the lung muscles, increased mucus production, increased permeability of the lung's blood vessels with weeping of serum into the tissue, and irritation of the lung's nerves, which produces cough. Thus the reaction in the lung to an allergen is analogous to the intestine's reaction to a parasite. This type of reaction, because of its rapid onset within 5 to 30 minutes after exposure to an allergen, is known as the *immediate response.* When a person allergic to a cat is exposed to cat dander, for example, symptoms develop within the first few minutes.

However, the allergic response does not end here. There is a second reaction, known as the *late phase response,* which occurs 2 to 6 hours after the immediate event. The late phase response is induced by an invasion of the lung by an army of cells, led by the eosinophil, called to the site by chemotactic agents released from the mast cell during degranulation. The cells then turn their internal arsenal of weapons against the allergen (seemingly viewing it as a parasitic invader) as they degranulate. The chemicals released from the cells damage the lung, and wheezing and shortness of breath recur (fig. 3.3).

The late phase response is more profound and prolonged than the early phase response, and sets up an ongoing process that has the capacity to damage the lung permanently if it continues. In addition, this type of chronic inflammatory response makes the lung more sensitive to *all* substances known to precipitate wheezing <diagram I>. Thus exposure to an allergen can enhance the lung's sensitivity to the other factors known to produce asthma, such as weather conditions, respiratory irritants (e.g., cigarette smoke), and exercise. This enhanced and exaggerated response is known as *bronchial hyperreactivity.* The degree of bronchial hyperreactivity correlates with the severity of asthma, and bronchial hyperresponsiveness varies over time. When the bronchial hyperresponsiveness is increased, the disease becomes more severe; when it is decreased, there is usually a lessening of symptoms. In addition, those who demonstrate the most bronchial responsiveness are as a rule the most severe asthmatics. Thus, we see the following chain of events:

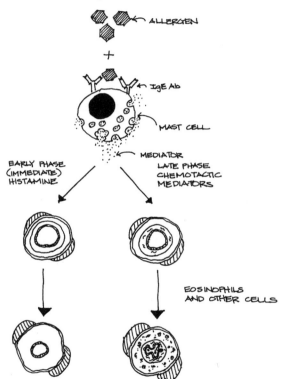

FIG. 3.3. The immediate and late phase allergic reactions. The immediate reaction occurs within minutes and is due to the direct effect of the chemical mediators released from the mast cell on the muscle, blood vessels, mucus glands, and nerves of the bronchioles. The late phase response is delayed a few hours and is due to the influx of cells, especially the eosinophil, to the lung. These cells are attracted to the site by chemicals released by mast cell degranulation. The influx of these produces the inflammation characteristic of asthma.

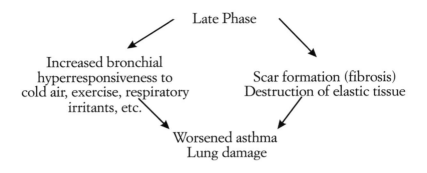

1. The allergen is inhaled.

2. The allergen unites with the allergic antibody that is affixed to the mast cell.

3. The mast cell degranulates, releasing its chemicals.

4. The chemicals cause, within minutes, contraction of smooth muscle, leakage of fluid into the lung, irritation of the cough nerve, and swelling of the bronchial tube. This, in turn, causes coughing, wheezing and shortness of breath.

5. Within hours, cells, especially eosinophils, travel to the lung, where they produce another response characterized clinically by coughing, wheezing, and shortness of breath that is more profound. This second reaction, known as the late phase response, in turn increases the bronchial hyperresponsiveness and has the potential to damage the lung permanently over a long period of time.

6. An increased bronchial hyperresponsiveness makes asthma worse on a daily basis and enhances the response to nonallergenic stimuli (such as irritants and weather conditions) that produce symptoms.

7. Finally, continuation of this type of activity over long periods of time can produce permanent damage with lung scarring.

Although this paradigm refers to allergy, a similar series of events occurs in the nonallergic asthmatic. There is evidence for mast cell degranulation in the nonallergic asthmatic (although it does not appear to be due to IgE antibody and allergen interaction), and nonallergic asthmatics also have a prominent eosinophilic invasion of the lung. In addition, on biopsy exam all of the changes noted in the allergic asthmatic are found in the nonallergic asthmatic as well.

Control of the late phase response is essential to the prevention of worsening of asthma and the potential long-term permanent tissue destruction that can occur with this illness. The mechanisms by which the late phase response are controlled will be discussed in chapter 5.

## Inheritance of Allergy

The exact nature of the inheritance pattern regarding allergy has not been established, but we do know with certainty that this condition runs in families. If one parent is allergic, the chance that each child will be allergic is approximately 33 percent. If both parents are allergic, the chance that each child will be allergic is approximately 50 to 70 percent.

The basic immunologic characteristics associated with allergy appear very early in life, perhaps even in utero; the ability to make IgE occurs in utero as early as eleven weeks. Children destined to be allergic manufacture larger amounts than those who do not have this genetic trait. In addition, the lymphocyte profile of such children is the one associated with allergic disease as described earlier (the TH2 prototype). The exact location of allergy-determining genes is not yet known. One resides on the same chromosome as the genes for IL-4 and IL-13 (the cytokines that enhance IgE production), IL-5 (the cytokine that enhances eosinophil proliferation), and the enzyme that produces leukotrienes. It is tempting therefore to think of this area as a prime site for the transmission of allergic diseases. However, other allergy genes have been identified in certain families, and probably many more will be.

# Nonallergy Triggers of Asthma

*From what I have heard from others, and as is known
to Your Highness, I conclude that this disorder starts
with a* common cold, *especially in the rainy season, and
the patient is forced to gasp for breath day and night,
depending on the duration of the onset, until the phlegm is
expelled, the flow completed and the lung well cleared. . . .
You also remarked that* strong winds *tend to hurt you
and* sharp smells *offend you much. Hair weighs on you
heavily and repeated shavings of the head brings you some
comfort. You wear no headdress and no turban, all of
which goes to show that your head suffers from excessive
heat. Your Highness has already confided in me that* the
air of Alexandria *is harmful to you and whenever you fear
an attack of the illness you prefer to move to Cairo where
the air is much dryer and calmer, making the attack more
tolerable for you.*

Moses Maimonides (1135–1204),
speaking to the son of Saladin,
the sultan of Egypt
(in *Treatise on Asthma*,
edited by Suessman Munter)

As we have seen, asthma is not a disease but rather a condition
with many triggers, allergy being one of the most, if not the
most, important. Allergy occupies this prominent role not only
because of the frequency with which it produces episodes and
the number of asthmatics afflicted with it, but also because

**Table 4.1** Nonallergy Triggers of Asthma

---

Upper respiratory tract infections (the common cold)

Exercise

Cold air

Irritants: Cigarette smoke, Air pollution, Perfumes, Aerosols,
   Paint fumes, Particulate dust

Associated medical conditions
   Rhinitis
   Sinusitis
   Gastroesophageal reflux

Medications
   Nonsteroidal anti-inflammatory drugs
   Beta-blockers

---

the allergic reaction serves as a model for the study of asthma. However, numerous other triggers of asthma exist as well (table 4.1).

## The Common Cold

The most important trigger other than allergy (in many patients an even more significant one) is upper respiratory tract infection, or the common cold. In fact, the common cold rivals, and perhaps exceeds, allergies, especially in adults, as a cause of hospitalization and death.

In the nonasthmatic, colds are usually simple nuisances characterized by spontaneously resolving symptoms usually lasting only 7 to 10 days. These symptoms include nasal congestion, runny nose, postnasal drainage, sore throat, swollen glands, and sometimes a feeling of fatigue. In some instances, the lower respiratory tract (bronchial tree) is also involved, and the nonasthmatic develops a bronchitis with cough. These symptoms can be confused with those due to allergies. In table 4.2 we can see the features that distinguish the common cold from upper respiratory tract allergies, an important distinction since many asthmatics suffer from allergies and often confuse the symptoms of a cold with those due to allergy.

All colds are caused by viruses. There are more than 240 viruses capable of causing the common cold, including the rhinovirus, coronavirus, influenza, parainfluenza, respiratory syncytial virus, adenovirus, coxsackie viruses, and echoviruses. Each of these major classifications of viruses contains many subclasses. The rhinovirus is the most common cause of colds and accounts for 30 to 40 percent of upper respiratory tract infections. The coronavirus accounts for up to 20 percent, and influenza, parainfluenza, respiratory syncytial virus, adenovirus, coxsackie virus, and the echovirus account for somewhere under 10 percent.

Colds are spread from person to person by direct contact and by aerosol. Direct contact can occur from individual to

**Table 4.2** Features that Distinguish Allergies from Colds (Upper Respiratory Tract Infections)

|  | Cold | Allergy |
| --- | --- | --- |
| Sore throat | Often | Almost never |
| Fever | Often | No |
| Green/yellow thick drainage | Usually after 2nd or 3rd day | Almost never |
| Sneezing | First 2 to 3 days | Yes |
| Itching eyes | No | Yes |
| Burning eyes | Occasionally | No |
| Swollen glands | Often | No |
| Occurring in winter | Yes | No, unless to pets |
| Occurring in spring/fall | Yes | Yes |

individual (shaking hands, kissing) or through the touching of a contaminated object. Direct contact is the most common form of transmission. Aerosol transmission via sneezing or coughing occurs less frequently.

Some of us are more at risk than others for the development of colds. Susceptible persons include adults who work around children (teachers and those employed in daycare centers), children who are in daycare and nursery school, people who frequently travel by airplane, and people involved in providing health care. The reasons for increased susceptibility are obvious. Transmission occurs more readily with greater exposure, as would occur in a daycare or elementary school setting. This is probably why mothers (who are more often the predominant care givers) have a slightly higher rate than fathers. Frequent air travel is a risk factor not only because of the close quarters but also because of the recirculated air.

Colds tend to occur seasonally; in fact, each virus seems to have its own season. The influenza epidemic (flu actually being the most severe form of cold) occurs annually, beginning in late fall and ending in early spring. The other cold viruses have similar recurring seasons, and many of us tend to redevelop our colds at the same time each year. This annual recurrence mimics allergy because it often coincides with the typical allergy fall and spring seasons.

As noted, most colds are self-limited and result in no significant illness. However, complications from colds that can occur in anyone, asthmatic or not, include bacterial infections such as infections of the sinuses and middle ear (sinusitis and otitis). In addition, severe upper respiratory tract infections producing bronchitis can lead to bacterial pneumonias.

Nonetheless, in the vast majority of instances, colds are simply nuisances. To the asthmatic, however, they can cause severe illness and even death.

The common cold, especially the version produced by the respiratory syncytial virus, is often, in children, the event that precipitates the onset of asthma. In addition, the onset of allergy per se is frequently initiated by these infections. For example, shortly after viral infections in childhood the susceptible child begins to manufacture allergic antibody and to experience allergy symptoms for the first time. Thus, these infections are not only precipitants of acute events but in some way seem to alter the immune response to initiate the development of allergy.

The precise means by which upper respiratory tract viruses precipitate asthma attacks is unknown; however, there are several possible mechanisms (table 4.3).

The first possible mechanism has been termed the "innocent bystander" effect. In such a case, the inflammatory effect produced by the virus on the lung causes swelling and mucus secretion. When the virus attacks the lung, it invades the cells lining the bronchi. These cells, known as *epithelial cells*, are infected by the virus; they die as a result of this invasion and are sloughed into the bronchial lumen. Then, since the cells themselves serve to transport mucus from the lower to the upper bronchi, mucus pools in the lumen of the bronchi. Also, because the cells are sloughed, the underlying tissue weeps. The weeping occurs because the epithelial cells form a protective layer over the "skin" of the airways. The loss of this protection

**Table 4.3** Mechanisms by which Viral Infections Cause Asthma

"Innocent bystander" effect—the direct inflammatory effect of the virus, causing narrowing of the airways

Loss of protective effect of the lining (epithelium) of the bronchi
  Loss of protective effect of epithelial secretions that destroy neuropeptides
  Loss of epithelial barrier protecting nerve endings

Virus acting as allergen

Enhancement of the release of chemical mediators from mast cells is analogous to skin being scraped from the external surface of the body. The fluid weeping from the underlying tissue is partly composed of serum and is viscous. The combination of pooling respiratory secretions and viscous fluid produces a tenacious mucus which is difficult to clear. In addition, cells rush to the lung. During the battle, inflammatory mediators are released which cause inflammation of the bronchial tissue. The tissue itself then swells. The cumulative effect of the excess secretions, thickening of the bronchioles due to the influx of cells, and swelling of the bronchioles from inflammation narrows the airway lumen. Thus the body's defense against infection and the resultant inflammation adversely affects the bronchi, which are in this instance simply "innocent bystanders."

The loss of the epithelium can cause asthma in other ways as well. Epithelium serves several functions, one being to manufacture enzymes known as *neutral endopeptidases.* These enzymes destroy chemicals known as *neuropeptides,* which are manufactured by the nerves that run from the brain to the airways. They are produced in excess by these nerves during times of inflammation. They contract smooth muscle and increase blood vessel permeability resulting in the leakage of serum into the airways. With the loss of epithelium and the resultant decline in production of neutral endopeptidases, these neuropeptides can exert their activities without control.

The epithelium also has another protective function, serving as a barrier lining that overlies and protects the endings of the nerves carrying messages from the lung to the brain. After receipt and interpretation of these messages, the brain responds and sends return messages to the lung. This process is a form of reflex and occurs at a subconscious level. The "lung-brain-lung" reflex is analogous to the pain reflex that communicates signals from the skin to the brain and back. For example, if we place our hand on a hot stove, an involuntary response occurs, resulting in the almost instantaneous withdrawal of our hand from the hot surface. This does not require a thoughtful decision but happens automatically. The most superficial layer of the skin is also composed of epithelial cells similar in function to those lining the inner surface of the bronchi. If skin cells are scraped, the pain nerve fibers are exposed and the skin then becomes overly sensitive when stimulated. Thus normally innocuous stimuli might result in these nerve fibers sending a message to the brain that would be interpreted as pain and result in withdrawal from the stimulus. This automatic withdrawal is produced by contraction of muscle. However, there are no pain fibers in the bronchi, and, obviously, the lung, trapped within the chest cavity, cannot withdraw from a noxious stimulus. Instead, the message that the brain sends back to the lung results in a constriction of the bronchial tubes and a contraction of the muscles of the chest and diaphragm, producing a cough that expels the cause of the irritation. In the skin this set of events is known as the pain reflex and in the lung as the cough reflex, and, since it results in constriction of the bronchial tubes, it is also known as the *broncho-constrictive reflex*. When the epithelium is denuded, reflex bronchial constriction is activated more easily since the nerve endings are exposed. Thus, viral infections enhance the broncho-constrictive reflex (fig. 4.1). The concept of reflex bronchospasm is important, since it also plays a role in asthma aggravated by sinusitis and rhinitis, as we will see later.

The virus can also act as an allergen. IgE antibody (the allergic antibody) is synthesized against the viral antigen. This IgE, uniting with the virus, then results in the degranulation of mast cells with the resultant release of histamine and other chemical mediators (see chapter 3).

Finally, viruses have the ability to enhance the release of chemical mediators from mast cells through other mechanisms. That is, after a viral infection, mast cells more easily release their chemicals when exposed to other agents such as pollen allergens. The dose of the pollen allergen required to degranulate mast cells is reduced after viral infections.

The cumulative effect of all of these events is not only a worsening of asthma during the infection but also a prolonged increase in bronchial hyperresponsiveness. After a viral upper

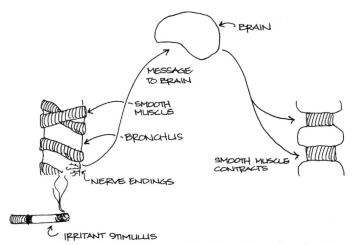

FIG. 4.1. The broncho-constrictive reflex. Stimulation of the lung's nerves sends a message to the brain, which results in a return message to the muscles of the bronchi causing them to contract, thus narrowing the airway.

respiratory tract infection, asthma is worse for many days or for weeks. The threshold of response to nonspecific agents such as cold air, exercise, cigarette smoke, or paint fumes is lowered. The asthmatic then becomes "more asthmatic" for a relatively prolonged period of time, usually several weeks, even though the infection itself has been conquered by the body.

It is important to realize that asthma episodes due to viruses can be not only severe but also sudden in onset. Lower respiratory tract symptoms of coughing, wheezing, and shortness of breath can occur within 24 hours after the onset of upper respiratory tract viral symptoms such as runny nose and nasal congestion. In fact, on occasion, wheezing can occur without any premonitory upper respiratory tract warning. Thus the asthma sufferer must be alert to the earliest onset of chest symptoms and to the premonitory upper respiratory tract symptoms that usually precede them. It is clear that early treatment, especially with oral corticosteroids (discussed in chapter 5) can prevent the often serious asthmatic consequences of the common cold.

It is therefore imperative that patients be able to recognize early warning signals.

## Exercise

Virtually all asthmatics wheeze with exercise. On occasion, individuals wheeze *only* with exercise. Quite often "exercise asthma" is a harbinger of full-blown asthma, which begins later in life.

Exercise asthma is produced by aerobic activity and can result from activities such as running, cycling, rowing, and swimming. The exercise must be fairly vigorous; asthma does not occur until a person's respiratory rate and heart rate are considerably elevated.

During the first 2 to 3 minutes of exercise, the bronchi dilate in nonasthmatics as well as in asthmatics. If exercise is continued over several more minutes, however, an asthmatic's bronchial tubes begin to contract, and towards the end of the exercise period lung function begins to degenerate further. The major bronchial constriction occurs within 5 to 10 minutes after exercise is stopped. Normal function of the lungs does not return until 30 to 40 minutes after the cessation of exercise. Usually, the more vigorous the exercise, the more intense the constriction of the bronchi and therefore the more severe the symptoms.

The major cause of exercise-induced asthma is hyperventilation, the production of rapid air flow through the bronchi. In fact, the bronchial constriction that occurs during exercise can also be induced by hyperventilation even in the absence of vigorous physical activity.

There are several hypotheses as to why the act of hyperventilating causes bronchial constriction, resulting in wheezing and shortness of breath. The exact mechanism has not been established, but two factors appear to play a role: the cooling of the airways and the evaporation of water from the airways surface that occur due to hyperventilation. The body's response to cooling is to rush more blood to the bronchial tubes for warmth, which is thought to engorge the blood vessels in the bronchi. The engorgement itself produces swelling and a reduction in size of the airway lumen. The evaporation of water from the surface of the airways produces not only cooling but also what is known as a hyperosmolar environment at the surface of the bronchi. Osmolarity refers to the concentration of particles in a fluid. As liquid evaporates from a fluid, the relative concentration of particles to liquid is increased. An above-normal particle-to-liquid ratio is referred to as hyperosmolarity. This can be viewed as a form of local dehydration. A hyperosmolar state of the fluid bathing the airways will result in degranulation of mast cells living in the airways. This degranulation is similar to that which occurs during the allergic response (see chapter 3) and results in the release of histamine, leukotrienes, and other substances by the mast cell. Thus, exercise can cause a reaction similar to the allergic response.

Because exercise asthma is produced by cooling and drying of the airways surface, it is more likely to occur when exercise is conducted in cold air and when there is little humidity. Thus exercise on a cold, crisp winter morning is more likely to produce wheezing than similar activity on a warm, humid day.

Some exercises are more likely than others to cause asthma, running being the most "asthmagenic," followed by cycling and then swimming. The exact reason for this hierarchy is unknown, but it is presumed that swimming causes less asthma because the swimmer constantly breathes in humidified air.

This kind of asthma can almost always be controlled, and asthmatics should be encouraged to exercise. It is usually advisable for a person to try to prevent exercise asthma by employing a medical regimen before the activity is undertaken. The most effective drug is an inhaled, rapid-acting beta-agonist (see chapter 5) used 30 minutes before exercise. If this agent alone is insufficient to control symptoms, other drugs can be added. Cromolyn sodium, nedocromil sodium, theophylline, and antileukotrienes (see chapter 5) are all effective agents for the management of this condition.

In addition, control of underlying chronic asthma reduces the patient's sensitivity to exercise.

## Irritants

Tobacco smoke is probably the most important indoor irritant known to cause asthma. This is a particularly poignant problem in children who have no control over their environment. It is quite clear that exposure to sidestream smoke is associated with significantly lowered levels of pulmonary function, the need for increased medication, absences from school and work, and a diminished quality of life in asthma sufferers. Moreover, pregnant women who smoke create a risk factor for the development of asthma in their children.

It has always been evident that air pollution exacerbates asthma. For example, exercise undertaken during periods of high pollution has been shown to cause more severe exercise asthma than similar activity occurring on days of less pollution. A number of air pollutants provoke symptoms, the most important probably being sulphur dioxide. High levels of nitrogen dioxide also correlate with increased emergency room visits and hospitalizations.

Indoor air pollutants may also play a role. For example, dust and perhaps sulphur dioxide produced by fireplaces can cause asthma symptoms. Nitrogen dioxide generated by gas heating may also cause problems.

Strong odors such as those from perfume, paint fumes, and cleaning agents can produce wheezing, as can dust that is stirred up on a drive down a gravel road.

Exactly how wheeze is produced by irritants is unknown; however, it is believed that these substances cause reflex bronchoconstriction by stimulating the nerve endings of the bronchi.

## Associated Medical Conditions

Three associated medical conditions—rhinitis, sinusitis, and gastroesophageal reflux—can aggravate asthma.

*Rhinitis* refers to inflammation of the nose; the symptoms are sneezing, runny nose, nasal congestion, and postnasal drainage. *Sinusitis* occurs, often as a complication of rhinitis, when the sinuses (cavities in the head surrounding the nose and connected to it via canals) become infected. Infection usually occurs due to nasal obstruction that blocks the canals connecting the sinuses to the nose and results in the accumulation of secretions in the sinuses, which then become infected by bacteria. Rhinitis can be caused by allergies or upper respiratory tract infections, or can occur chronically in the nonallergic individual (chronic nonallergic rhinitis), a condition analogous to nonallergic or intrinsic asthma.

It is unclear how rhinitis and sinusitis adversely affect asthma, but the worsening is believed to be due to reflex bronchoconstriction. That is, the brain receives messages from the nerves of the sinus and nose which are then in some way confused with messages it receives from the nerves of the lungs. Interpreting the messages from the nose and sinuses as if they were coming from the lungs, the brain sends back messages to the lungs resulting in bronchoconstriction.

There are other, perhaps more well-known, examples of "confused messages" occurring in the body. For example, heart attack victims often feel pain not in the area of the heart but down the left arm or at the angle of the jaw, the brain having interpreted the message as coming from somewhere other than the heart.

It has been shown that treatment of rhinitis and sinusitis can reduce the severity of asthma.

*Gastroesophageal reflux* occurs when acid from the stomach gains access to the swallowing tube, or esophagus. It is commonly known as "heartburn." A valve at the junction between the esophagus and stomach normally prevents reflux of acid from the stomach into the esophagus; when this valve becomes weakened, such reflux occurs. Reflux is clearly aggravated by asthma per se, since the lungs are hyperexpanded, which puts pressure on the stomach and increases the potential for reflux. Coughing creates further pressure, exacerbating the problem. Finally, many of the drugs that we use to treat asthma (oral beta-adrenergic agents and theophylline) relax the sphincter separating the stomach from the esophagus, further worsening reflux. Thus, not only does reflux worsen asthma, but asthma and its treatment aggravate reflux.

There are two possible mechanisms by which the reflux can intensify asthma: a reflex bronchoconstriction (similar to that for sinusitis and rhinitis) and the inhalation of stomach contents. The reflex is initiated by acid getting into the esophagus. Once again, as with rhinitis and sinusitis, this process titillates a nerve ending, which sends a message to the brain that is often confused with messages originating in the lungs. The brain then sends a message back to the muscles surrounding the bronchi of the lungs to contract. This is another form of reflex bronchospasm.

Acid reflux may also exacerbate asthma due to the fact that small amounts of stomach contents can be inhaled, especially during sleep. The acid then irritates the lung lining, causing reflex bronchospasm and producing an inflammatory reaction.

Thus it is important for asthmatics to control esophageal reflux, and there are several medications which are highly effective in this regard. These include forms of antihistamines that block the formation of stomach acid, which histamine stimulates. Examples of this class of drug are cimetidine (brand name Tagamet), ranitidine (Zantac), nizatidine (Axid), and famotidine (Pepcid). Histamine causes gastric acid production, and these drugs, by blocking the action of histamine, reduce gastric acid secretion. Another class of agents, even more effective in reducing gastric acid production, are the proton pump inhibitors. (The proton pump exchanges hydrogen [acid] for potassium in the lumen of the stomach, thus increasing gastric acidity.) These drugs include lansoprazole (brand name

Prevacid) and omeprazole (Prilosec). Another medication, cisapride (Propulsid), enhances the emptying of the stomach into the intestine, thus decreasing the chance that stomach contents will flow into the esophagus. Finally, the medication metoclopramide (Reglan) assists the function of the sphincter separating the esophagus from the stomach and thereby can reduce reflux. These medicines are usually highly effective in controlling reflux. Other measures that do not involve medication can also be employed to reduce gastroesophageal reflux (table 4.4).

**Table 4.4** Ways to Reduce Gastroesophageal Reflux

---

Eat several small meals rather than a few large ones. Large meals put pressure on the stomach and increase the amount of reflux.

Avoid exercise or lying down for at least two hours (preferably three) after eating.

Do not eat within three hours of bedtime.

Avoid clothes that constrict the waist.

Elevate the head of the bed 6 to 8 inches (wood blocks can be used). This helps gravity work to prevent reflux.

Maintain a healthy weight. This is extremely important. Those who are overweight should reduce. The more weight there is around the abdomen, the more pressure there will be on the stomach, causing an increase in reflux.

Do not smoke.

Avoid certain foods that seem to aggravate the problem. Any food or drink containing caffeine or a related substance can increase reflux; these include chocolate, coffee, tea, and caffeinated cola drinks. Many patients seem to be affected by spicy foods and some by peppermint.

Consider medications (see text) if symptoms are not controlled by these measures.

---

## Medications

Some asthmatics are particularly sensitive to aspirin and all drugs in its family, which are used to treat pain and arthritis and are known as nonsteroidal anti-inflammatory drugs (NSAIDs). Several of these (aspirin, naproxen, ibuprofen, ketoprofen) are available over the counter and many others by prescription (table 4.5).

It is not known how common nonsteroidal anti-inflammatory drug sensitivity is in asthmatics. In various reports, frequency is given from 3 percent all the way to approximately 40 percent of asthmatic adults. It is far less common in asthmatic children.

Most, but not all, aspirin-sensitive asthmatics have other associated problems, including sinusitis, severe rhinitis, and nasal polyps. *Nasal polyps* are benign inflammatory growths, with roots in the sinuses, which protrude into the nostril. The

**Table 4.5** Some Nonsteroidal Anti-inflammatory Drugs*

aspirin (acetylsalicylic acid) (Bufferin, APC, Excedrin, Anacin)

diclofenac sodium (Voltaren)

fenoprofen calcium (Nalfon)

ibuprofen (Motrin, Rufen, Advil, Nuprin)

indomethacin (Indocin, Indocin SR)

ketoprofen (Orudis)

meclofenamate sodium (Meclomen, Meclofen)

naproxen (Naprosyn)

naproxen sodium (Anaprox)

piroxicam (Feldene)

sulindac (Clinoril)

tolmetin sodium (Tolectin)

*Generic terms are lowercased; brand names are capitalized.

occurrence of sinusitis with nasal polyps, aspirin sensitivity, and asthma has been known as the *aspirin sensitive triad*. Any asthmatic who has nasal polyps and chronic sinusitis should avoid the ingestion of nonsteroidal anti-inflammatory drugs. It should be noted, however, that the first manifestation of the aspirin sensitive triad can be a reaction to aspirin, with the sinusitis and polyps occurring later in life. Thus the absence of sinusitis and nasal polyps does not automatically rule out the presence of nonsteroidal anti-inflammatory drug sensitivity.

Why asthmatics have nonsteroidal anti-inflammatory drug reactions has been studied extensively. Although there is some debate as to the exact mechanism, we do understand the fundamental nature of this type of adverse event. The key molecule involved is a substance known as arachidonic acid, which is present in the membranes of cells. It is normally fixed in place in the membrane, but any type of inflammatory stimulus can release it from its moorings. Any form of damage to the membrane such as that occurring in arthritis, asthma, or even physical trauma cleaves arachidonic acid from the membrane. At that point it enters the body of the cell (cytoplasm) and is subsequently metabolized by two pathways. One of these pathways, the cyclooxygenase pathway, produces prostaglandins, which do many things, including increasing pain sensitivity. For example, they are associated with the pain of arthritis and of physically traumatic events such as dental work. The other pathway is the lipoxygenase pathway, which results in the formation of leukotrienes. (As we saw in chapter 3, leukotrienes are chemical mediators that can cause asthma.)

Aspirin inhibits the formation of prostaglandins. That leaves more arachidonic acid available for the lipoxygenase pathway and the production of leukotrienes, which can result in exacerbations of asthma. In addition, some prostaglandins prevent the degranulation of mast cells. When their production is diminished, mast cells will degranulate more easily. Finally, leukotrienes can enhance the degranulation of mast cells. Thus, after an asthmatic who is sensitive to nonsteroidal anti-inflammatory drugs ingests one of these agents, there is not only increased production of leukotrienes but also increased release of histamine and other agents from mast cells.

Drugs known as beta-blockers (beta-adrenergic blocking agents) are useful in treating a number of conditions, including high blood pressure, cardiac arrhythmias, glaucoma (when given by eye drops), and migraines, and in the prevention of heart attacks. The beta-adrenergic system refers to the neurologic system, which relaxes the smooth muscle of the bronchial tree and stimulates the heart. Blockage of this system can, while calming the heart, constrict the muscles of the bronchi. This broncho-constrictive tendency occurs in an exaggerated form in asthmatics, who should, when at all possible, avoid beta-blocking drugs.

# Controlling the Condition

*In all grave disorders marked by seizures, such as lum-*
*bago, inflammation of the joints, gravel (in the kidney),*
*asthma (also called shortness of breath), migraine,—in*
*all of them, provided the prescribed regimen is well kept*
*and judiciously applied, the intervals between two onsets*
*may be lengthened, the duration of the onset so shortened*
*and its intensity mitigated. However, should the rules of*
*management go unheeded and one's desires and habits*
*be followed indiscriminately, the gap between onset will*
*grow shorter, and the duration and intensity gradually*
*increase until a peak is reached . . . The six obligatory*
*regulations are: (1) keeping clean the air which we breathe;*
*(2) keeping an eating and drinking diet; (3) regulation of*
*spiritual emotions; (4) regulation of bodily exercise; and*
*lastly rest (5) sleep and waking up; (6) excretion, even-*
*tually keeping back the superfluous outflow. The seventh*
*group is the one the body takes according to circumstances,*
*such as bathing and massaging.*

Moses Maimonides, *Treatise on Asthma*

Although we do not yet know the cause of this affliction, we
have come a long way since Maimonides, a medieval physician,
philosopher, and rabbi, gave advice to the legendary sultan
Saladin and cared for the Muslim leader's son. Today, as a
result of our increased understanding of the mechanisms of

production of asthma, we are able to control, although not cure, this condition adequately in the vast majority of those afflicted. This is possible because of knowledge gained through basic investigation. The treatment of asthma is an excellent example of the application of knowledge gained at the "bench" (that is, through basic scientific research) and used at the "bedside" (in the patient's life).

Three broad categories of therapy exist for asthmatics. Two of these, *environmental control* and *allergen immunotherapy*, apply solely to the allergic asthmatic. The third, *symptomatic control with medication*, applies to all asthmatics regardless of type.

Each of these types of therapies will be discussed in detail, but first it is important to distinguish between what we call *disease modifying agents* and those which simply treat symptoms (referred to in this chapter, logically enough, as *symptom treaters*). Optimal care of all but the mildest asthmatics requires the use of disease modifying agents.

The concept of disease modification is a relatively new wrinkle in asthma therapy. Until the early-to-mid-1980s, when the scientific community reawakened to the role of inflammation, almost all medical care was directed at controlling the patient's symptoms. Thus far asthma had been thought of as a reversible disease, so that, if patients *felt* well, they were considered to *be* well. As we have seen, this concept has been revised based on more recently acquired information. We now know that an inflammatory process occurs even in asthmatics who are relatively asymptomatic and that it enhances the severity of the disease and can produce permanent damage, so the current focus is not only to control symptoms but also to modify that process. The tools of therapy that have the potential of modifying the disease process will be referred to in this chapter as disease modifying agents. These agents can also control symptoms and make the patient feel better, but their major function is to reduce the severity of the disease by controlling inflammation and to prevent permanent lung damage.

It might be helpful to look at another kind of situation in which medications are used. If someone has a brain tumor, for example, the only manifestation might be pain. If the pain is controlled, the patient is unaware of any potential damage to the brain from continued expansion of the tumor. But even though the person feels fine, the tumor may be expanding and damaging surrounding brain tissue. In this case a disease modifying agent would be one that actually shrank the tumor so that no damage would occur. The patient is unaware of it, but in fact is much healthier than if the tumor's expansion were not being controlled.

A similar situation exists in asthma. The patient may feel well because symptoms are being controlled with a medication that keeps the bronchial tubes open, but the disease could be progressing, producing lung damage and an increase in bronchial hyperresponsiveness that might result in more profound attacks at a later date. Agents that simply control the constriction of the bronchi in an asthmatic would therefore be analogous to agents that only control pain in the patient with the brain tumor, hiding the manifestations while allowing the disease to go unmodified.

Disease modifying agents are in essence drugs with anti-inflammatory effects; that is, they tend to reduce the inflammatory process in the lung produced by the influx of cells. By doing so they dampen the late phase response as discussed in chapter 3 and also reduce bronchial hyperresponsiveness as well as the potential for permanent lung damage. Symptom treaters, however, fail to reduce the inflammatory response and therefore have no effect on either bronchial hyperresponsiveness or the potential for long-term permanent lung damage. The benefits of disease modifying agents may not be apparent to the sufferer because they do not provide the dramatic, immediate effects that make the patient feel better quickly, as symptom control agents would. Thus, although the beneficial effects of disease modifying agents are well established, patients often underutilize them and overuse symptom treaters. Asthma sufferers should learn about disease modifying agents so as to be able to distinguish them from drugs whose major effect is only to control symptoms (table 5.1).

The National Institutes of Health Expert Panel Report of 1997 makes these distinctions quite clear; however, the discussion in this book is somewhat different from the one in the 1997 guidelines. In this chapter, drugs are divided into *disease modifiers* and *symptom treaters*, whereas, in the guidelines, agents are described as "quick relief medications" and "long-term controller medications." Quick relief medications are

**Table 5.1** Asthma Treatments Classified as Symptom Treaters and Disease Modifiers*

| Symptom Treaters | Disease Modifiers |
|---|---|
| *Beta-adrenergic drugs* | *Corticosteroids* |
| albuterol (Proventil HFA, Ventolin) | Oral (e.g., prednisone, |
| bitolterol (Tornalate) | methylprednisolone) |
| metaproterenol sulfate (Alupent) | Inhaled |
| pirbuterol acetate (Maxair) | beclomethasone (Beclovent, |
| salmeterol (Serevent) | Vanceril) |
| terbutaline sulfate (Brethaire) | fluticasone (Flovent) |
| | triamcinolone (Azmacort) |
| *Theophylline* | flunisolide (AeroBid) |
| (e.g., Theo-24, Theo-Dur | budesonide (Pulmicort) |
| Uniphyl) | |
| | *Nonsteroidal anti-inflammatory drugs* |
| *Anticholinergic drugs* | cromolyn (Intal) |
| ipratropium bromide (Atrovent) | nedocromil (Tilade) |
| | *Antileukotrienes* |
| | zafirlukast (Accolate) |
| | montelukast (Singulair) |
| | zileuton (Zyflo) |
| | *Environmental control* |
| | *Allergen immunotherapy* |

*Generic terms are lowercased; brand names are capitalized.

drugs that are used for immediate symptom control but have no anti-inflammatory activity. Thus they are all symptom treaters. However, some of the long-term controller drugs mentioned in the guidelines do not have significant anti-inflammatory activity and are therefore *not* disease modifying. They are called long-term controllers only because they must be used on a regular basis rather than "as needed only" in order to be effective. They share this feature with disease modifiers, which are also taken regularly. In the 1997 guidelines, "long-term controllers," regardless of whether they are disease modifiers or symptom treaters, are all classified together only because each must be taken regularly. The patient must be able to distinguish long-term controllers with anti-inflammatory activity from those without such activity. Examples of long-term controllers without anti-inflammatory activity are the long-acting beta-agonist drugs such as salmeterol and sustained release tablets of albuterol as well as theophylline. This distinction is mentioned so that the reader can avoid confusion with the classification noted in the National Institutes of Health guidelines, which is becoming a standard reference source.

Drugs that have very little anti-inflammatory activity (symptom controllers) are known as "bronchodilating" agents; that is, they relax the smooth muscle surrounding the bronchioles and thus enlarge the airway diameter. They do produce excellent relief of symptoms but have very little effect on the influx of the inflammatory cells, and therefore do not lessen bronchial hyperresponsiveness or protect against lung scarring. The three categories of such agents are beta-adrenergic agents, theophylline, and anticholinergic agents.

Drugs that affect inflammation, on the other hand, have only modest bronchodilating activity. They include corticosteroids, cromolyn sodium, and nedocromil. A new class of agents, antileukotriene drugs, have modest-to-moderate bronchodilating activity and seem to be anti-inflammatory as well. These drugs will be discussed individually later in this chapter.

In the allergic asthmatic, environmental control measures (avoidance of allergen) and allergen immunotherapy (allergy injections) have anti-inflammatory effects and can reduce bronchial hyperresponsiveness. The mechanisms underlying the activity of these therapies will also be discussed later in this chapter.

Thus, disease modifying agents appear to have activity on the late phase, bronchial hyperreactivity and perhaps on long-term lung damage, while symptom-treating drugs have their major effect, and perhaps the only significant one, on the contraction of the smooth muscles surrounding the bronchi and therefore on the early phase reaction.

We can use the model of asthma discussed in chapters 2 and 3 to look at these agents and contrast their activity (fig. 5.1). A summary of the effects of these drugs, employing the asthma paradigms discussed earlier, is shown in table 5.2.

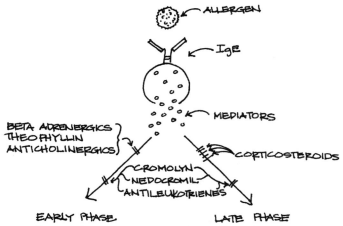

FIG. 5.1. Effects of therapeutic agents on the early and late phase responses of the allergic reaction.

Agents with potential disease modifying activity can have a modest-to-moderate effect on the early phase response (bronchoconstriction due to smooth muscle contraction) if

**Table 5.2** Characteristics of Disease Modifying Agents and
Symptom Treating Agents

|  | **Disease Modifying Potential** | **Symptom Treating Agents** |
|---|---|---|
| Effect on early phase response | With some agents, under certain circumstances | Yes, very good; beta-adrenergics the most effective |
| Effect on late phase response | Yes | No |
| Effect on inflammation | Yes | No |
| Effect on bronchial hyperresponsiveness | Yes | No |
| Effect on permanent damage | Possibly | No |

given before the inhalation of allergen; they have very little
effect if given afterward. For example, both cromolyn sodium
and nedocromil can prevent the early phase response if given
before allergen inhalation. Inhaled corticosteroids given for
many weeks before allergen inhalation can also reduce the
early phase response to a modest extent. Oral corticosteroids
given days to hours before the inhalation of allergen can blunt
the early phase response to some extent. The same is true for
antileukotriene agents. However, by far the most profound effect
on the early phase response is achieved through the activity of
the bronchodilating agents—that is, agents that relax smooth
muscle. The most effective of these are the beta-adrenergic
agents. Theophylline is also somewhat helpful in this regard, and
anticholinergic agents, through a different mechanism of action,
can also modify the early phase response to some extent.

In contrast, only agents with anti-inflammatory activity
(those with disease modifying potential) have an effect on the

late phase response. These include corticosteroids, cromolyn sodium, nedocromil, and antileukotriene agents. Long-acting beta-adrenergic agents and theophylline can mask one of the manifestations of the late phase response (continued contraction of smooth muscle) but do not actually alter this response to any great extent (although there is some evidence that theophylline can do so modestly).

It is logical to assume, since the late phase response is due to inflammation, that only those drugs that affect the late phase response will have a significant effect on inflammation. Indeed, this is the case. Once again, corticosteroids, cromolyn sodium, nedocromil, and probably the antileukotriene agents have an effect in this regard, whereas the bronchodilating agents (beta-adrenergics and theophylline) do not to any great extent (although, again, there is some evidence that theophylline might have a very modest effect).

Since bronchial hyperresponsiveness, which, as we have seen, is an index of the severity of the disease, is in great part related to the late phase response and inflammation, drugs that affect the late phase response and inflammation will reduce bronchial hyperresponsiveness, whereas those which are smooth muscle relaxants (beta-adrenergic agents and theophylline) do not.

It is thought that permanent damage is related to the presence of inflammation, so it would be logical to assume that those drugs which have anti-inflammatory potential could prevent permanent damage. Thus far, however, there are no definitive studies documenting the effect of anti-inflammatory agents on long-term lung damage, although there is evidence that topical (inhaled) corticosteroids as well as cromolyn and nedocromil can have a salutary effect in this regard.

Specific allergy therapy—allergy injection and environmental control—does not constitute medication per se but nonetheless should be evaluated according to the same criteria as those for drugs. Allergy injections have been shown to affect both the early and late phase response as well as to decrease bronchial hyperresponsiveness. However, their effect on inflammation has not been extensively evaluated. Allergen avoidance, on the other hand, reduces bronchial hyperresponsiveness considerably. For example, it has been shown that individuals allergic to house dust mites, when removed from exposure to the mite, exhibit a marked reduction not only in their response to dust mite inhalation challenge but also in what is known as their nonspecific bronchial hyperresponsiveness (response to the inhalation of cold air, respiratory irritants, methacholine, and exercise). Thus specific allergy therapy should be considered as disease modifying.

We can therefore appreciate that the principles of application of asthma therapy modalities are based upon a knowledge of the basic inflammatory nature of the disease. Such treatment modalities are then divided into those which exert anti-inflammatory activity and those whose major effect is simply to open the airway by relaxing the smooth muscle surrounding it. Each particular agent has its own characteristics, however, and a knowledge of these is important for the asthma sufferer.

## Drugs

### Drugs with little or no anti-inflammatory reactivity (symptom treaters)

*Beta-adrenergic agents* can be taken by inhalation, by mouth, or by injection. These agents exert their primary effect by relaxing the smooth muscle that surrounds the bronchial tubes. They do this by stimulating a receptor on the smooth muscle, which then sends a message instructing the cell to manufacture a substance known as cyclic AMP that in turn produces relaxation through a complicated series of biochemical events. They are by far our most effective bronchial muscle relaxing medication. The 1997 guidelines divide these agents into "quick reliever" and "controller" categories. The reliever category consists of inhaled drugs that cause onset of action within minutes. They should be used *only as needed for acute relief*, and are known as *rescue drugs*. Because these drugs are never used on a regular basis, the need for one is an excellent indicator of the severity of the illness—that is, the smaller the need, the less active the condition. Noting the number of puffs per day taken on a rescue inhaler is useful in determining the necessity for other agents and in warning the patient of an impending attack. Whenever the patient has to use these inhalers for more than 2 to 3 puffs per 24 hours, it is a sign that additional measures should be taken to control the asthma. These drugs, as noted, have no anti-inflammatory effect.

Beta-adrenergic agents are also available for long-term symptom control (not anti-inflammatory control). There is a long-acting inhaler known as salmeterol which exerts its activity over a 12-hour period. On the other hand, salmeterol does not produce an immediate effect, as do the rescue beta-adrenergic inhalers such as albuterol and pirbuterol. It should never be employed on an "as needed only" basis. An alternative to the use of salmeterol is a long-acting oral beta-2 adrenergic agent such as a sustained release oral albuterol preparation.

As noted, none of the beta-adrenergic agents exerts any significant anti-inflammatory activity, but they are the best drugs for the relief of acute symptoms. The major side effects of beta-adrenergic drugs are irritability, jitteriness, insomnia, tremors of the hand, and fast heartbeat. In most instances these side effects are minimal, and quite often patients develop tolerance to them over time.

*Theophyllines* are related to caffeine (found in coffee and cola drinks) and theobromine (found in tea). In fact, it has been shown that coffee and tea exert a modest bronchial dilating effect due to caffeine and theobromine. Theophyllines act in much the same way beta-adrenergic agents do, in that their major effect is to relax the smooth muscle surrounding the bronchial tubes, which causes them to dilate. The precise means by which theophylline exerts its effect has not been established, but it can act through what are known as adenosine receptors on smooth muscle surfaces. In addition they can prevent the destruction of cyclic AMP (a chemical that can relax the smooth muscle of the bronchi). Their immediate bronchial dilatory effect is probably mediated through the adenosine receptor, whereas long-term effects may be the result of their prevention of the degradation of cyclic AMP.

Unlike beta-adrenergic agents, theophyllines are no longer "as needed" agents used to control acute attacks. They are administered only by mouth (except during acute asthma, when they are occasionally given intravenously), and therefore their onset of action is slower than that of inhaled, rapid-acting beta-2 adrenergic agents. At this time they are used almost entirely as maintenance drugs, administered by mouth on a regular basis to prevent asthmatic episodes. However, because of several disadvantages, use of this class of drug in the United States has decreased over the last decade. With overdosage or with the administration of drugs that prevent the metabolism of theophylline in the liver, profound side effects such as seizures and heart arrhythmias can occur. Lesser side effects including nausea, irritability, and insomnia also occur quite often. In order to prevent these side effects, many patients must have their blood levels of theophylline measured, which entails additional costs and inconvenience. With the recent availability of inhaled long-acting beta-adrenergic agents and antileukotriene drugs, which can be just as effective with fewer side effects, the use of theophylline in its present form will probably continue to decline. However, on the horizon is a new generation of theophylline-like preparations which are more selective for lung smooth muscle and therefore cause fewer side effects. Perhaps in the future these theophylline-like drugs will produce a renaissance in the use of this class of agent.

*Anticholinergic agents* are not approved by the Federal Drug Administration (FDA) for treatment of asthma. They are used mainly in other obstructive bronchial diseases such as emphysema and bronchitis. However, in some asthma patients they are effective adjuncts to beta-adrenergics and/or theophylline, because they work in an entirely different way.

Instead of dilating smooth muscle by a direct action on the muscle itself, they block the activity of the vagus nerve, which produces a chronic, constant physiologic contraction of the smooth muscle of the lung. The vagus nerve also carries the message from the brain that mediates reflex bronchoconstriction (see chapter 4). Anticholinergics therefore reduce the small amount of chronic muscle contraction present constantly and modulate reflex bronchoconstriction, so that their effect is often additive to that of beta-adrenergics and theophylline. In addition, they may play a special role in certain asthmatics who are taking drugs that block the activity of beta-adrenergic agents. Such drugs, known as beta-adrenergic blockers (see chapter 4), are administered to individuals with migraines, cardiac arrhythmias and other diseases of the heart, and high blood pressure. In some instances, their administration is essential, and they cannot be discontinued. In patients with asthma who require beta-adrenergic blocking agents, an anticholinergic agent such as ipratropium (brand name Atrovent) is an extremely useful bronchodilator since it does not act through the same mechanism that beta-adrenergic drugs do. In addition, anticholinergic drugs are useful in the therapy of the acute asthmatic episode. There are few side effects related to the administration of anticholinergic drugs by inhalation.

### Drugs with anti-inflammatory (potentially disease modifying) activity

*Cromolyn sodium* and *nedocromil* are called, for lack of a better term, *nonsteroidal antiinflammatory asthma agents*; they exert anti-inflammatory activity similar to that produced by corticosteroid drugs but are not themselves corticosteroids. (This name is somewhat misleading, since these agents are in no way related to the drugs discussed in chapter 4 that are used to treat arthritis and pain.) The advantage of using them is that anti-inflammatory activity is produced without the development of any of the side effects that occur with corticosteroid administration. As a rule, these agents are not as effective as corticosteroids in the control of symptoms or in the modification of inflammation; however, there is little doubt that they do control inflammation, and some evidence exists that they can reduce the potential of long-term lung damage.

These agents seem to work in nonallergic asthmatics but appear to have a far more potent effect in those with allergies. Their mechanism of action is incompletely understood, but it is clear that they have several biological effects. One of these is the prevention of degranulation (release of chemicals including histamines and leukotrienes) from mast cells. The means by which this is accomplished is unknown, but it is believed to be related to the fact that these agents prevent the entry of chloride into cells by blocking what are known as chloride entry channels. Chloride passage into the cell is essential for some inflammatory activities, such as mast cell degranulation, and for the transmission of nerve impulses from the lung to the brain to mediate reflex cough and bronchospasm. These drugs have other effects such as slowing the travel through nerves that carry cough impulses.

These agents must be administered on a regular basis. For the most part, they have beneficial effects only when used before the inhalation of allergen or exposure to other stimuli known to be asthmagenic. They are effective not only in allergen-induced asthma but also in preventing symptoms due to exposure to respiratory irritants such as sulphur dioxide and cold air. In addition, they are effective in the prevention of exercise-induced asthma.

These drugs are almost totally devoid of significant side effects, although coughing does occur, and some individuals have difficulty with the taste of nedocromil.

Neither agent has bronchodilating activity.

*Antileukotriene drugs* are another agent in this category. As we saw in chapters 2 and 3, leukotrienes are chemical mediators that are manufactured in eosinophils and mast cells and that are released in large amounts during exacerbations of asthma.

They are also produced chronically in smaller (but significant) amounts on a constant basis in the asthmatic. Thus they are in part responsible for some of the chronic constriction of bronchial muscle that many asthmatics experience on a constant basis. It is not surprising therefore that the administration of these drugs produces a modest bronchodilating activity by antagonizing the constantly present broncho-constrictive effect due to chronic leukotriene production. However, their bronchodilating activity is not the most important therapeutic effect of this class of drugs. In addition to producing smooth muscle relaxation, they also can reduce the influx of eosinophils into the lung, decrease bronchial hyperreactivity, decrease mucus secretion, and prevent the activation and proliferation of fibroblasts (thus, theoretically, the laying down of ground substance). Therefore these drugs appear to have anti-inflammatory activity as well.

Three antileukotriene drugs are available in the United States—zileuton, zafirlukast, and montelukast. Zileuton blocks the synthesis of leukotrienes, whereas montelukast and zafirlukast block the activity of leukotrienes at their cell receptor sites.

Even though these drugs do exert a modest bronchodilating activity (similar to that of theophylline, for example), they are not to be used on an "as needed" basis as are rapid-acting beta-adrenergic agents but are to be taken on a regular basis for prevention of symptoms.

Almost no serious side effects accompany these drugs. One of the agents, zileuton, can produce abnormalities in liver function, so when this drug is administered the patient's liver function should be assessed periodically. Neither zafirlukast nor montelukast has been associated with significant liver function abnormalities; therefore, their use does not require a blood test measuring liver function activity. Zafirlukast interacts with other drugs such as blood thinners, and there is some indication that it might also interact adversely with theophylline. At the time of this writing, no such drug interaction has been demonstrated for montelukast.

*Corticosteroids* are the most potent anti-inflammatory drugs in our therapeutic arsenal and are by far are the most effective agents for the management of asthma. They can be administered by mouth, by inhalation, and by injection.

A revolution in asthma management occurred in the 1970s with the introduction of inhaled corticosteroids that exert little systemic effect. These drugs have, perhaps more than any other agent, improved the quality of life for patients with moderate and severe asthma. Most such patients require corticosteroid management (at least intermittently) for control. In the past, before the availability of inhaled corticosteroids, the only means of administration was by mouth or injection. Since these forms of systemic administration can produce profound and sometimes disabling side effects, the availability of inhaled agents, which are in many cases almost equally effective for maintenance therapy and which do not produce such effects, has been a boon for the asthmatic sufferer.

Since oral corticosteroid therapy is now almost totally limited to the treatment of acute exacerbations, these drugs are classified, in the 1997 guidelines, as relievers. However, they differ from relievers such as rapid-acting bronchodilators in that they are slower in onset (usually they do not exert obvious benefit until 1 to 2 hours after ingestion) and in that they exert their beneficial effect through anti-inflammatory activity rather than via bronchial dilatation. They are far more potent than bronchodilators in the control of acute exacerbations.

Inhaled corticosteroids exert no immediate effect but are used as preventive agents; they are taken daily on a regular basis.

The exact mechanism of action of corticosteroids is unknown. We do know that they act at the cellular level to cause cells to decrease their production of asthmagenic substances and perhaps increase the production of substances which reduce inflammation. Unlike other drugs, which act through cell surface receptors, corticosteroids diffuse into the cell and bind with a receptor within the cell itself (cytoplasmic receptor). From there they are transported to the nucleus, where they turn off inflammatory agent genes and turn on anti-inflammatory agent genes. In the test tube, new production is noticed within 20 minutes, but in the asthma sufferer, as noted, activity of systemic corticosteroids takes at least an hour and usually longer.

Unfortunately, systemically administered corticosteroids (oral or injection) can cause profound side effects when given over a long period of time (months to years). These include cataracts, glaucoma, softening of the bones (osteoporosis), a predisposition to diabetes with elevation of the blood sugar, thinning of the skin with easy bruising, weight gain with deposition of fat around the abdomen, cheeks, and back of the neck, and slowing of growth in children. While short-term administration does not produce these serious side effects, lesser but sometimes very bothersome ones can occur, including jitteriness, irritability, fluid retention, insomnia, and flushing. The short-term side effects that some patients (although certainly not all) experience are being hot, red, swollen, irritable, and unable to sleep. In spite of these side effects, more severe asthmatics often require the administration of systemic corticosteroids at least intermittently, and, rarely, a patient requires systemic administration on a regular basis.

In contrast to systemic corticosteroids, inhaled corticosteroids do not cause serious side effects to any great extent, because major activity occurs at their site of deposition in the lung, and they are absorbed only in small amounts. In addition, most of these agents are metabolized very rapidly in the liver. However, it is clear that this systemic absorption, even though modest, can produce side effects, although to a less extent than in systemic administration. The most prominent of these are thinning of the skin with easy bruising, a tendency towards early formation of cataracts and glaucoma, some degree of bone softening (at least upon measurement of chemicals in the blood that are related to such softening), and slowing of growth in children. But these effects are usually not clinically significant. Less threatening local side effects are more common. These occur due to the local deposition of corticosteroids on the tissues of the mouth and throat and include a predisposition to fungal infections in the mouth (commonly known as thrush) and a weakness of the muscles controlling the vocal cords, which produces hoarseness.

Nonetheless, the side effect/benefit ratio of these drugs clearly favors their use. The inhaled corticosteroids, more than any other agents, have improved the management of asthma and the quality of life for the asthmatic patient. In addition, there is evidence that these agents can prevent long-term lung damage.

*A schema for the employment of*
*medications in the therapy of asthma*

The most widely adopted format for the employment of these agents is contained in the 1997 *Guidelines for the Diagnosis and Management of Asthma*. The therapy employs a stepwise approach, since drugs are added (and deleted) in such a fashion depending upon the severity of the illness in an individual sufferer. There are four categories (stages) of severity: mild intermittent, mild persistent, moderate persistent, and severe persistent. Table 5.3 shows the characteristics of each group and indicates the drugs used in the treatment of each step. As the illness worsens, drugs are added in a "step-up" fashion, and, as the illness abates, drugs are diminished in a similar "step-down" fashion.

Several features of this format deserve comment. One of the most important new recommendations is the very early use of what is called a controller agent, which is advocated in patients with symptoms occurring more than two times a week (that is, who have to use a short-acting rescue beta-adrenergic agent more than twice a week), and/or those whose asthma awakens them from sleep more than two times a month (stage II, mild persistent asthma). In the past, asthma of this severity would have been considered extremely mild, and a controller agent would not have been administered. However, because of the recognition that inflammatory activity occurs very early on in asthma and the observation that quality of life can be

**Table 5.3** Classification of Asthma Severity

| | Symptoms | Nighttime Awakenings | Drugs |
|---|---|---|---|
| Step I Mild intermittent | Brief episodes occurring less often than twice a week | Less often than twice a month | Use rapid-acting inhaled symptom reliever only (e.g., albuterol). |
| Step II Mild persistent | Symptoms occurring more often than twice a week but less often than daily | More often than twice a month | Add anti-inflammatory disease modifying agent, preferably low dose inhaled corticosteroid, cromolyn, or nedocromil. Antileukotriene may be appropriate (see text). |
| Step III Moderate persistent | Daily symptoms that affect activity, some episodes lasting days | Once a week or more | Increase dose of inhaled corticosteroid and add additional agents such as long-term symptom relievers (salmeterol, theophylline). May also add antileukotriene if not presently taking. |
| Step IV Severe persistent | Continual symptoms that limit physical activity with frequent exacerbations | Frequent | Multiple drugs are often required. Inhaled corticosteroids should be raised to maximally recommended dosages. Oral corticosteroids are often necessary. |

improved with the early institution of controller therapy, the guidelines promulgate the use of controllers at an early stage in relatively asymptomatic individuals. It should be pointed out that the controllers recommended by the guidelines at this stage are not all anti-inflammatory or disease modifying agents. The guidelines give the option of adding inhaled corticosteroids in low doses, cromolyn or nedocromil, an antileukotriene agent, or a sustained release theophylline preparation. As noted, it is doubtful that sustained release theophylline has any significant disease modifying effect, and thus its use at this stage is difficult to justify. The use of an antileukotriene agent at this stage is debatable only on the grounds that we have little experience with these drugs to date. On the other hand, there is at least strong theoretical evidence that these agents are anti-inflammatory, which means that their use at this stage is more easily justifiable than the use of theophylline. However, the "tried and true" anti-inflammatory agents (inhaled corticosteroids, nedocromil, and cromolyn), at least at the time of this writing, are preferable.

Stage III, moderate persistent asthma, is characterized by the presence of daily symptoms requiring the use of a short-acting beta-agonist, by exacerbations of the illness that affect the patient's activity and that last for days, and by asthma-induced interruption of sleep once a week or more. At this stage, patients usually require at least intermittent systemic corticosteroids and inhaled corticosteroids in medium doses. Also at this stage, an antileukotriene, a long-acting beta-2 agonist such as salmeterol, and/or a sustained-release theophylline may be indicated.

It should be clear that the guidelines are, as their name states, *only* guidelines. These recommendations should not be accepted as dogma; there are still "many ways to skin a cat" in asthma therapy. But they do provide a format and certainly give insight as to an expert panel's perception of the nature of the disease and the therapy required.

## Allergen Avoidance

It is crucial for allergic individuals to avoid allergens. The presence of allergic sensitivity is best determined by a medical history and confirmed by allergy skin testing. When the results of skin testing confirm a history of allergen-induced exacerbations, the diagnosis of allergic asthma is established. One of the most important concepts regarding reduction of allergen exposure is that it not only prevents a particular allergen from producing symptoms but can also reduce nonspecific bronchial hyperresponsiveness. That is, avoidance of allergen exposure can also reduce the severity of symptoms caused by other asthma triggers such as cold air, exercise, cigarette smoke, and weather conditions. The proposed rationale for this reduction in nonspecific bronchial hyperresponsiveness is that reducing exposure to allergens will in turn decrease the inflammatory process in the lungs by preventing mast cell degranulation due to allergen inhalation. The reduction in inflammatory response will make the sufferer "less asthmatic" and lead to a reduction in episodes produced by other exposures.

It is also important to note that for many patients removal of an allergen can "cure" the illness. While the disease and the potential to experience it are not truly eliminated, patients may show such a marked reduction in symptoms that they no longer require therapy. This is often the case when asthma is caused by exposure to an indoor pet; when the animal is removed from the home, the patient becomes totally asymptomatic after a few months and no longer requires medication. Allergen reduction can be accomplished for animal danders, dust mites, pollen, and, to a lesser extent, cockroaches and molds. A typical allergen avoidance protocol is shown in table 5.4.

## Immunotherapy (Allergy Injections)

Allergen immunotherapy is the injection of allergens to which the patient is sensitive and which therefore cause symptoms.

**Table 5.4** Environmental Control Measures

---

**House Dust Mites**     The bedroom, the most important room in the house as far as environmental control is concerned, should be kept well dusted and vacuumed (twice a week is usually standard). Dusting should be done with a commercial preparation that picks up dust. When dusting and vacuuming, those with allergy should wear a pollen mask, which can be obtained at a drugstore. The mattress, box springs, and usually the pillow should have allergy covers, which can be purchased at department stores. The air conditioning filter should be changed every 2 to 3 months. The bed linen should be washed on the "hot" cycle in the machine so as to kill dust mites.

**Grass Pollen**     People allergic to grass pollen should avoid yard work, especially mowing, if they can. Those who must do yard work should wear a pollen mask.

**Indoor Pets**     Most people with allergies are allergic to animals; thus they should not, in general, have indoor pets. Outdoor pets are fine as long as they do not come into the house. It is imperative that allergic asthmatics not have indoor pets, since this condition is potentially serious. Unfortunately, simply keeping pets out of the bedroom is of little help.

**Feathers and Down**     Comforters, mattresses, and pillows should not contain feathers or down.

---

These injections are given in gradually increasing doses until amounts usually a million times stronger than the initial dose have been reached. Through this regimen, the immune response to the allergen is altered and a type of tolerance to the inhalation can be achieved. Allergen immunotherapy is usually administered over a three-to-five year period. Initially injections may be given on a weekly basis, and, after the first year and a half to two years, a gradual reduction in frequency is undertaken. Patients usually take injections once every other week for six months to a year, once every third week for six months to a year, and then once every fourth week for six months to a year.

Allergen immunotherapy may improve symptoms of asthma related to allergen inhalation. It is indicated when there is clear evidence of a relationship between the symptoms and exposure to an unavoidable allergen such as pollen, especially when there is difficulty in controlling symptoms with medication or when there are side effects from it.

Studies have shown that allergy injections have been helpful in controlling symptoms due to the inhalation of tree, grass, and weed pollen, dust mites, and certain mold spores.

The mechanism of action of allergen immunotherapy has not been conclusively established. However, it is clear that the injection of allergen produces an immune response that is radically different from the one produced by inhalation of allergen as described in chapter 3, and a number of unique immunologic effects occur during the administration of immunotherapy (table 5.5 and fig. 5.2).

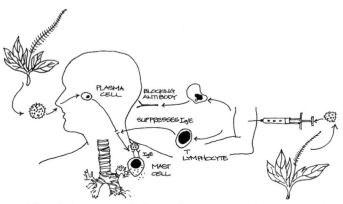

FIG. 5.2. The administration of allergen by injection induces immunologic changes that cause a shift to the $TH_1$ profile, produce blocking antibodies, and decrease the production of IgE.

One of the earliest observed immunologic effects of immunotherapy was the production of what has been called "blocking antibody." The name derives from the fact that this

**Table 5.5** Some Immunological Effects of Allergen Immunotherapy for Asthma

---

Production of "blocking antibody"

Decrease in IgE antibody to allergen
    Long term
    Postseasonal

Changes in T-Cell Profile
    Generation suppressor T-cell
    Shift from TH2 to TH1

---

antibody, known as IgG, can compete with the allergic antibody, IgE, for allergen. In certain experimental systems, IgG antibody, by binding allergen, can prevent its union with IgE and thus diminish the intensity of the allergic response. The level of blocking antibody does show a rough correlation with the degree of symptom relief in large groups of individuals treated with allergen immunotherapy. However, this correlation is imperfect; some individuals with high levels of blocking antibody get little relief, whereas others with low levels obtain excellent relief.

Blocking antibody appears not only in the bloodstream but also in the secretions. When present in the secretions, it often consists of a different class of antibody known as IgA.

In addition to the production of blocking antibody, allergic antibody levels tend to decline with long-term administration of allergen immunotherapy. This was first demonstrated over 30 years ago with the observation that allergen skin test reactivity can be reduced by the long-term administration of allergy injections. The effect was rediscovered as a result of the development of techniques to measure IgE antibody against specific allergens. In addition to the long-term decline in IgE antibody, there is a blunting of what is known as the postseasonal rise in IgE. Normally, production of IgE antibody against an allergen increases during the allergy season. Allergy injections can prevent that increase.

The mechanism responsible for the reduction in IgE production has not been elucidated, but it is probably due to changes in the T-cell profile. As we have seen, T-cells are the conductors of the immune response. There are two main types, effector T-cells and regulatory T-cells. Regulatory T-cells comprise helper and suppressor T-cells (see chapter 3). Helper cells assist in the synthesis of IgE antibodies, and suppressor cells exert the opposite effect. During immunotherapy, specific suppressor T-cells are generated against the allergen used for therapy. It is thought that these suppressor T-cells are responsible for the decline in IgE antibody that occurs with treatment. There is a shift from the T helper cell 2 to the T helper cell 1 profile. As discussed earlier, the T helper cell 2 profile is characterized by the production of interleukins that enhance IgE production (IL-4 and IL-13) and increase the survival and activity of eosinophils (IL-5). On the other hand, TH1 cells produce gamma interferon, IL-2 and IL-12. IL-12 can diminish the production of IgE.

These immunologic effects have clinical consequences in that both the early and late phase response to allergen challenge can be blunted by allergen immunotherapy, which in turn can reduce bronchial hyperresponsiveness. So in some ways this therapy can be considered anti-inflammatory in nature.

To summarize, in this chapter we have discussed therapies, their mechanisms of action, and the rationale for their use based upon the classification of asthma severity. Therapeutic agents have been divided into those with potential disease modifying (anti-inflammatory) activity and those which affect symptoms only. We have learned how these agents are used in asthma therapy according to the severity of the disease. We have seen that it is important to establish an anti-inflammatory or disease modulating regimen early on even when the disease is considered mild. We have also noted that, for the allergic asthmatic, environmental control is an extremely important aspect of therapy, as is, in some cases, allergen immunotherapy.

Finally, we have seen how important it is for the asthmatic to understand the basic mechanism of action of each agent employed in treatment and also how these agents are classified according to effect. Lack of such understanding can result in a progression of the disease and will certainly diminish quality of life for the sufferer.

# Tools of the Trade

*On auscultation, with inspiration and expiration, there are innumerable sibilant and sonorous rales of all varieties, piping and high pitched, low pitched and grave.*
Sir William Osler, *The Principles and Practice of Medicine*, 1884.

The "sibilant . . . rales" and other sounds mentioned by Sir William Osler describe what was heard through the stethoscope. With that being the only tool available then, detailed description and analysis of sounds were important in establishing a diagnosis. The stethoscope itself was invented by René Théophile Hyacinthe Laënnec in 1814. For approximately the next 100 years it was the only device physicians had for the evaluation of the asthmatic. We now have sensitive and accurate instruments with which to assess the severity of the illness and establish the diagnosis. We also have tools designed to assist in treatment.

It is, of course, not necessary for the asthmatic to have a detailed knowledge of the mechanisms by which such instruments accomplish tasks, but familiarity with the tools themselves is useful.

## Pulmonary Functions

Asthmatics, unfortunately, are often unable to assess the severity of their illness on the basis of symptoms. They are notoriously inaccurate in assessing the degree of air flow obstruction caused by bronchial tree narrowing. And physicians, using the techniques of physical exam including the stethoscope, are no more accurate. Thus there is a need for objective assessment of lung function. This is particularly important in the assessment of function during an acute episode and in serial assessments of function over long periods of time.

We have two techniques for the objective assessment of airway flow. One of these, the *peak flow rate*, can be performed at home by the patient with a portable device known as a *peak flow meter* (fig. 6.1). The other, *spirometry*, is employed in the physician's office. Spirometry is more sensitive and accurate and gives more information, but the peak flow meter is still extremely useful for home monitoring.

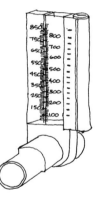

PEAK FLOW METER

FIG. 6.1. Peak flow meters are small, portable devices that give objective measurements of air flow.

Both of these devices measure the rate of air flow through the bronchial tubes. The peak flow measures, in liters of air per minute, the highest speed of air obtained during a forced expiration. Spirometry measures not only the peak expiratory flow but also the maximal volume of air the patient is able to expire, the rate of expiratory air flow during the first second of expiration, and the rate of expiratory air flow during the middle portion of expiration. The rate of expiratory air flow during the first second of expiration is the most important of these values.

For each of these tests, the patient inhales deeply and then expires into the device employed. To measure a peak flow, the patient "explodes" air into the device as rapidly as possible. It is not necessary to empty the lungs entirely for a peak flow measurement. The aim of the peak flow measurement is to detect the most rapid rate at which air can flow through the lungs. On the other hand, during spirometry, the patient not only breathes air out as fast as possible but also must empty the lungs by exhaling to a maximal extent.

During an asthma attack the peak flow rate is reduced. Patients can set their normal peak flow—that is, their personal best—by performing the peak flow maneuver while they are without symptoms. Then, should they develop symptoms, the peak flow rate is used to assess the severity of the episodes objectively. Some patients underestimate their attacks, and in this case a peak flow measurement is essential to prevent serious episodes. In other instances, episodes of shortness of breath not due to asthma (when air flow is not slowed) can be distinguished from those due to asthma (when air flow is slowed) to help establish the diagnosis of asthma when it is in doubt. Peak flows have additional uses as well. They can determine whether or not asthma is due to a specific exposure, which is important in assessing whether or not asthma is related to an occupational situation, for example. The peak flow can be taken while individuals are at work and also while they are at home, so that they can determine whether differences in air flow exist at the two places.

Peak flow readings are traditionally divided into zones. These zones are based on either the normal value (peak flow normal values are based on age and height) or the patient's personal best value (when the patient has chronic irreversible disease and is never able to reach a normal value). Peak flow "zones" are then set according to the degree of airway obstruction, reflected by a reduction in peak flow. For example, 80 to 100 percent of the normal or personal best value is considered a "safe" zone, or within normal limits. Mild obstruction occurs when the value is between 65 and 80 percent of normal or personal best, and moderate obstruction when the value is 50 to 65 percent of normal or personal best. A value of below 50 percent indicates a severe episode.

Peak flow can also act as a surrogate for more sophisticated means of measurement of the degree of airway hyperresponsiveness. As we have seen in previous chapters, airway hyperresponsiveness means that there is increased reactivity of the asthmatic bronchioles to external stimuli such as cold air or respiratory irritants. This increased sensitivity is manifested by sudden contraction of the smooth muscle surrounding the bronchi, which produces obstruction to air flow and, naturally, a fall in peak flow. The degree of hyperresponsiveness can be measured and quantified by a test known as a methacholine challenge, in which the asthmatic is asked to inhale gradually increasing doses of methacholine, a chemical that causes smooth muscle contraction. The asthmatic is far more responsive than the nonasthmatic to this chemical. The degree of responsiveness correlates directly with the severity of the illness. As a rule, the more hyperresponsive an asthmatic is to methacholine, the more severe the disease. Peak flow measurements can be used as a substitute for a methacholine inhalation challenge test. This is done by measuring the difference between the morning peak flow (obtained when the patient arises from sleep) and the evening peak flow (obtained at bedtime). The morning peak flow is usually lower than the evening peak flow, a difference known as the diurnal variation. Mild asthmatics have a diurnal variation in peak flow of less than 20 percent, mild persistent asthmatics usually have a variation of between 20 and 30 percent, and a variation greater than 30 percent is consistent with moderate or severe asthma.

Thus people with asthma can gain much information from serial measurements of peak flow. First of all, they learn to correlate their subjective assessment of the severity of the illness with an objective measurement, which is a form of biofeedback training. The peak flow can also give an early warning of an impending attack. Patients can assess the variability of their bronchial hyperresponsiveness and thus the state of their asthma by serially determining the diurnal variation in peak flow. The effects of medicines on this diurnal variation can also be monitored. Information as to what might affect asthma can also be gained by a monitoring of the peak flow. For example, peak flow measurements might be correlated with weather conditions (humidity, a front coming in) or with exposures (cigarette smoke, perfume). Peak flow measurements can also be used as guides for the addition or deletion of medications to or from the treatment regimen.

It is important to know that peak flow measurements depend upon technique, and the correct technique is crucial. The peak flow should be measured three times, and the highest value should be used. Maximal expiratory effort is required. Patients should avoid placing their tongues against the peak flow mouthpiece before exhaling. (A detailed description of the proper use of the peak flow meter can be obtained from any one of a number of organizations listed in the appendix.)

Finally, one practical point regarding the measurement of peak flows is that the readings between different peak flow meters vary considerably. The patient's personal best will vary depending upon the type of commercial peak flow meter purchased; thus each time a new peak flow meter is obtained, the normal or personal best must be reset.

A pulmonary function study performed in the physician's office gives additional information in a more sensitive and accurate manner. The physician may use a pulmonary function measurement to assess the response to drugs, measure the severity of a given episode, or trace lung function over long periods of time to assess whether or not there is evidence of permanent lung damage. Objective assessment of pulmonary function is recommended even for mild asthmatics on an annual basis and for more severe asthmatics at least twice to three times per year.

## Metered Dose Inhalers

Metered dose inhalers are used to deliver aerosolized drugs to the lung. As with peak flow meters, their correct use requires careful attention to technique. Improperly used, these agents will fail to deliver the drug to the bronchi.

One metered dose inhaler, the Maxair Autohaler, is self-actuated, which eliminates the need for close attention to the inhalation technique. When a patient puts the mouthpiece into his or her mouth and breathes in, a valve is activated and releases the medication. However, this is the only self-actuated inhaler available for use at the present time.

It is best for patients to review their use of metered dose inhalers periodically with their physician or a physician's assistant. Many studies have shown that, in spite of adequate instruction and proper initial usage, over time inhalation technique may degenerate; thus, periodic reviews are helpful. (See appendix for sources of instruction regarding proper inhalation techniques when a metered dose inhaler is used.)

## Spacer Devices

Some patients are unable to master the correct technique for inhalation and need help from a spacer device, which is designed to be connected to a metered dose inhaler at one end and to be put into the recipient's mouth at the other (fig. 6.2). The medication is then sprayed into the spacer and inhaled from this device. The spacer device serves several purposes:

1. It eliminates the need for perfect inhalation technique, which is required when the drug is delivered directly from the metered dose inhaler. The most common inhalation error occurs when the patient does not coordinate the release of medication

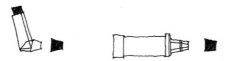

EXAMPLE OF SPACER #1

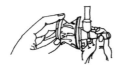

EXAMPLE OF ONE FORM OF SPACER #2

FIG. 6.2. Spacer devices assist in the delivery of inhaled drugs.

from the metered dose inhaler with inhalation. This is called actuation-inhalation discoordination. Faulty timing in this regard results in failure of the medication to be delivered to the lungs. Spacer devices of adequate size serve as holding chambers; that is, they hold the medication within the spacer chamber in aerosol form, thus allowing the patient to inhale the drug at a more leisurely pace and eliminating the necessity for actuation-inhalation coordination.

**2.** Spacer devices can increase the amount of drug delivered to the lung.

**3.** When spacer devices are used for the inhalation of corticosteroids, they can decrease the frequency of side effects due to deposition of the corticosteroid on the throat or larynx.

Thus, spacer devices should be used in almost all instances for the inhalation of corticosteroids and in any individual unable to coordinate inhalation and actuation regardless of the drug being delivered by metered dose inhaler.

Numerous spacer devices are on the market, and it is crucial to pick the one best designed to accommodate the drug being used. At this time the following matches are felt to be most appropriate: flunisolide (brand name AeroBid) is best administered through the Aerochamber and beclomethasone (Vanceril or Beclovent) through an InspirEase device. Triamcinolone (Azmacort) comes with its own self-contained spacer, which should be used. It is not currently known which spacer is best for fluticasone (Flovent).

A number of different dry powder inhaler devices are being developed which will eliminate the need for the special inhalation technique required for aerosol inhalation. These dry powder inhalers will make use of a different inhalation technique that is easier to master. Thus dry powder inhalation devices do not require a spacer. At present only one such device is available for the delivery of corticosteroids and two for the delivery of beta-adrenergic drugs. The corticosteroid dry powder inhaler delivers budesonide and is called a Turbuhaler. The dry powder inhalers for beta-adrenergic drugs are the Ventolin Rotacaps preparation and the Serevent diskus inhaler. Additional dry powder inhalation devices will probably become available in the future.

## The Eosinophil Count

As noted in previous chapters, the eosinophil is perhaps the most important effector cell in asthma. The number of eosinophils in the lung, as well as the number in the peripheral blood, increases with the activity of the disease, which means that these levels reflect the severity of an attack. Thus the measurement of a blood eosinophil count helps the physician assess the activity of the illness. Eosinophils travel from the bone marrow to the lung through the blood, and determining how many are present in the bloodstream during this journey gives an indication of whether or not the disease is in an active state. This test is extremely important in patients taking medications that control the symptoms. In such a patient the lung functions can be relatively normal while the disease itself can be active, since the drugs (such as inhaled corticosteroids) inhaled into the lungs control the manifestations of the illness but exert very little if any systemic effect. Thus the blood level of eosinophils is relatively unaffected by the medication. In this instance, knowledge of the number of eosinophils in the peripheral blood helps the physician in making the decision as to whether or not the dose of inhaled corticosteroids can be lowered. A low eosinophil count indicates that the disease is relatively inactive and that a reduction in medication would not result in an exacerbation. An elevated eosinophil count, on the other hand, can indicate disease activity and thus presage an exacerbation of the illness should the dose of medication be reduced.

## Methacholine or Histamine Challenge

As we have seen, asthma is characterized by a state of bronchial hyperreactivity, which can be measured by an assessment of the response of the bronchi (as determined by spirometry) to the inhalation of histamine or methacholine. This test is most useful in ruling out asthma as the cause of shortness of breath or wheeze. If the patient does not respond to the inhalation of methacholine or histamine, a diagnosis of asthma can be excluded. On the other hand, a positive test does not establish the diagnosis, since patients with other conditions, such as chronic bronchitis, can also be hyperreactive to the inhalation of these agents.

## Diffusion of Carbon Monoxide through the Lung

During pulmonary function testing, the diffusion of carbon monoxide from the air into the lung can be measured. The degree of diffusion depends upon the integrity of the air sacs (see chapter 2) and not on the state of the bronchi, so the diffusion of carbon monoxide in asthma is usually normal. On the other hand, the diffusion of carbon monoxide in emphysema (in which there is destruction of the air sacs) is abnormal. Thus this test can help the physician distinguish between these two illnesses, both of which cause shortness of breath.

## Allergy Testing

Allergy testing can be accomplished in two ways: through a skin test or a blood test. In the skin test, the allergen is either placed on the skin, which is then pricked, or is injected directly under the skin (fig. 6.3). In the blood test, the presence of IgE antibody against the allergen is detected by the incubation of the blood with allergen affixed to a solid surface (such as a test tube) and the addition to this blood allergen mixture of an indicator to detect the presence of IgE in the patient's serum. The IgE will be affixed to the test tube surface because it binds to the allergen (fig. 6.4). If the patient has IgE directed to the allergen, the IgE will bind to the allergen after the test tube is washed and unbound serum removed. Then an antibody against human IgE is added to the mixture. This antibody will bind to the patient's IgE at the end of the molecule opposite the one bound to allergen. The union of the patient's IgE with the antibody directed against it activates an indicator system. The indicator is attached to the antibody against IgE (opposite the end that binds to IgE). Thus a "sandwich" is formed, with the allergen (affixed to the solid surface) on one end and the indicator system on the other. Between the ends of the sandwich are the patient's IgE and the antibody against the IgE.

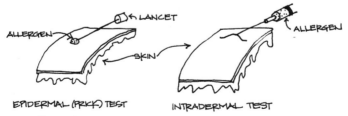

FIG. 6.3. Allergy skin testing.

The indicator system is usually based on the activity of an enzyme capable of producing a color change. This enzyme is attached to the antibody directed against the patient's IgE. The

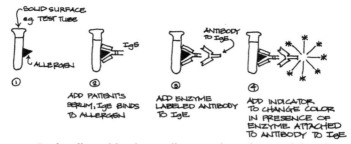

FIG. 6.4. In the allergy blood test, allergen is bound to a solid surface such as a test tube. The patient's serum is added to the tube. If the serum contains allergy antibody (IgE) to the allergen, the antibody will attach to the allergen and thus will be fixed to the wall of the tube. An "indicator antibody" can then be added to the test tube. The indicator antibody, which is directed against IgE, will attach to the patient's IgE. The amount of indicator antibody attached to the IgE can be quantified and will be proportional to the amount of the patient's IgE against the allergen.

enzyme is activated when this antibody binds to IgE, and the activation causes a color change which can be quantified. The degree of intensity of the color change is a reflection of the amount of antibody bound to the patient's IgE, which is in turn related to the amount of antibody bound to allergen.

Both the skin test and the blood test have advantages and disadvantages, but overall the skin test is the one of choice. Its advantages are: (1) it is read almost immediately, whereas the blood test is usually performed on a later date; (2) the reaction on the skin mimics the reaction in the lung, with a positive response showing redness, itching, and swelling, which gives the patient some insight as to the nature of the reaction in the lung; (3) it is more sensitive; and (4) per test it is less expensive.

The blood test is useful for those who cannot be skin tested (infants and people with generalized dermatitis).

So we have come a long way since Osler and his detailed description of sounds heard through a stethoscope, and, as we will see in the next chapter, the pace of progress is accelerating.

# A Look into the Future

*In recent experiments carried out in this laboratory . . .*
*evidence has been brought forward which indicates that*
*the contractions of smooth muscles caused by different*
*venoms are not their direct effects nor are they wholly*
*brought about by liberation of histamine. There is formed*
*from tissue constituents by enzymic action of the venoms*
*a "slow-reacting smooth muscle-stimulating substance"*
*which may largely determine the nature of these responses.*
*It was suggested that a similar mechanism might be in-*
*volved in the reaction of smooth muscles to other injurious*
*stimuli.*

Charles H. Kellaway and Everton R. Trethewie,
"The Liberation of a Slow-Reacting Smooth
Muscle Stimulating Substance in Anaphylaxis,"
*The Quarterly Journal of Experimental Physiology*, 1940

Charles Kellaway and Everton Trethewie were scientists
studying the effects of chemicals on the guinea pig intestine. The
above quotation is taken from their first description of a chemical
called slow-reacting smooth muscle stimulating substance (SRS).
In a laboratory far removed from asthma research per se, a
discovery was made that resulted in the awarding of a Nobel
Prize to an unrelated investigator 40 years later and in the
subsequent synthesis of a whole new class of compounds with
potent antiasthma activity. Kellaway's and Trethewie's SRS
turned out to be leukotrienes, perhaps the most important
chemical mediator of asthma.

The story of how this seemingly unrelated and isolated
finding (which was published in a journal not even read by most

physicians) evolved into one of the century's most important advances in asthma therapy is typical of scientific progress. Such progress is often initiated in laboratories devoted to basic research in the study of problems that originally have no obvious connection to the practical day-to-day management of disease. In this instance, Kellaway and Trethewie were out to show that chemicals other than histamine might play a role in producing the contraction of smooth muscle caused by cobra venom. The substance that they identified, which caused a more profound and prolonged contraction than histamine, initially failed to attract the interest of physicians dealing with asthma. In fact, more than 40 years passed before the exact chemical structure of SRS was identified (the discovery that led to the Nobel Prize) and the importance of this compound truly appreciated. The discovery of the identification of the structure of SRS resulted in a renaming of the molecule and the coining of the term "leukotrienes," and it also prompted the pharmaceutical industry to search for leukotriene antagonists, the result being the drugs mentioned in chapter 5 which are today improving the quality of life for asthmatics throughout the world.

This chapter is intended to give the reader a glimpse of present-day SRS-like research, which will, everyone involved hopes, one day have equally profound effects on the controlling of asthma. Some of this research does have a *Star Wars* aspect, being so futuristic that it is hard to visualize the potential practical benefit. But that was the situation in 1940 when Kellaway and Trethewie described SRS. Only the most imaginative could have foreseen the final result of that experiment conducted in a laboratory in Australia.

Advances such as the one initiated by the original description of SRS have, in the past 5 decades, revolutionized the care of the asthmatic. I first saw a patient with severe asthma in 1967. He was a 13-year-old boy who had spent almost his entire life institutionalized and who required the daily administration of oral corticosteroids (prednisone) to remain alive. The drug itself, given over a period of time, together with the ravages of asthma resulted in his premature death at age 17. At that time, the only other therapeutic agents we had were ephedrine, epinephrine, isoproterenol, and theophylline. Almost all of these have since been replaced by less toxic and more effective agents. The ensuing three decades have seen remarkable advances in our basic knowledge regarding asthma and its causes, which means vast improvement in the asthma patient's quality of life. An individual such as the young boy described above is almost unheard of today.

These advances are numerous, and mentioning a few will give the reader a flavor of the accomplishments. They include the discovery of IgE as the antibody responsible for allergic asthma and the delineation of its structure, the discovery of the receptor for IgE on the mast cell and the delineation of its structure, the aforementioned identification of the structure of SRS and many of the other mediators responsible for the production of asthma, the identification of the late phase response and its relationship to the production of chronic asthma, the establishment of the eosinophil as a primary effector cell in the illness, the development of the concept of bronchial hyperresponsiveness, the reawakening of the interest in inflammation in asthma, the identification of the TH1 and TH2 cells and their respective role in the illness, and the discovery of the role of upper respiratory tract viral infections in the production of asthma episodes. These basic discoveries have led to wonderful new therapies such as inhaled corticosteroids, more specific and less toxic bronchodilators such as the presently available beta-adrenergic drugs that act almost solely on the lung and do not stimulate the heart, cromolyn and nedocromil, and the antileukotriene agents. In fact, it is hard to remember what the situation was like when I first cared for an asthmatic.

It is not too farfetched to imagine that present-day research will result in equally effective advances in the future. In fact, with gene therapy in the wings and rapid progress in the search for responsible genes, it is even conceivable that we could eliminate this condition in the not-too-distant future.

The task of introducing readers to this research is somewhat difficult, because the basic science behind much of the work involves new disciplines that are at present far removed from the day-to-day affairs of asthma care, and which therefore can be foreign even to physicians specializing in the area. The research is being carried on in laboratories by individuals with expertise in the new sciences of molecular biology and molecular immunology, disciplines so new that they were not even taught during my training.

## Monoclonal Antibodies

Emil von Behring and Shibasaburo Kitasato were perhaps the first to realize the therapeutic power of antibodies. Working together at Koch's Institute for Infectious Diseases in Berlin in 1890, they injected a rabbit with tetanus and then withdrew blood from the rabbit and injected it into two mice. They described the protective effect of serum obtained from a rabbit immunized against tetanus: "Both animals [the two mice injected with serum taken from the immunized rabbit] . . . were inoculated . . . with virulent tetanus bacilli, sufficient to induce . . . death after 36 hours . . . Both pretreated mice remained healthy, throughout." This experiment gave birth to the use of antibodies for the treatment and prevention of infectious diseases. Antibodies were obtained from animals immunized with the infectious agent, and serum from these animals was collected and given to individuals infected with the disease. Thus were developed antisera against tetanus, diphtheria, rabies, and snake venom. However, there were two problems with this therapy. The first was that the production of antisera was tedious and expensive, requiring kennels of animals who were repeatedly immunized with the infectious agent. But, more important, the injection of animal antisera into human beings produced reactions in the recipients. The animal protein was recognized as foreign, and many recipients would develop either acute allergic reactions that were potentially fatal (anaphylaxis) or more slowly developing allergic reactions that were temporarily disabling (serum sickness). Thus therapy and prevention with antisera were limited in scope. This changed in 1975 when a technique for producing cell hybridomas was perfected. This technique ushered in the age of therapy with *humanized monoclonal antibodies*.

A *hybridoma* is a cell formed from the fusion of two separate cell lines that maintains characteristics of both. For the production of a hybridoma capable of manufacturing antibodies in large amounts, one of the cell lines must be obtained from an animal immunized with the substance (*antigen*). This animal will produce an antibody to the substance. The second cell line is obtained from a separate animal that has multiple myeloma, a form of cancer of antibody-producing cells known as *plasma cells*. Multiple myeloma cells, being from a cancer cell line, are "eternal" in that they will continue to reproduce indefinitely outside of the body when grown in appropriate cultures. Since they are cancerous antibody-producing plasma cells, they have the capability of manufacturing large amounts of antibodies. When this cell line is fused with the plasma cells obtained from the immunized animal, producing the desirable antibody, the end result is a progeny cell line with the following features: (1) eternal growth in culture outside of the body bestowed by the multiple myeloma cell; (2) ability to manufacture extremely large amounts of antibody, once again from the myeloma cell line endowment; and (3) ability to make antibody against the antigen administered to the immunized animal.

In this way, for example, plasma cells taken from a mouse immunized with tetanus can be fused with plasma cells taken from a mouse with multiple myeloma, producing a cell line that will manufacture large amounts of antibodies to tetanus for as long as it is grown in the laboratory.

Hybridomas solved one of the problems associated with the production of antisera obtained through immunization of animals; it was no longer necessary to maintain a large number of animals to which antigen was continually administered. Once a cell line was established, large amounts of antibodies could be harvested easily from the cultures. However, the second problem remained—the illnesses that occurred in the recipients of the antiserum as a result of the injection of animal protein. The antibodies grown in culture still were those of an immunized animal, in most instances a mouse.

That problem was solved with the development of antibody splicing techniques. As we have seen, the antibody molecule has two ends. One end combines with the antigen (the substance at which the antibody is directed—in this case the one against which the original animal was immunized), with the other end performing different functions. The portion that combines with antigen actually is only a very small segment of the antibody molecule. It was theorized that if this small segment could be removed and attached to a human antibody molecule, the human recipient would not recognize this new or spliced hybrid molecule as foreign. When technology became available to perform antibody splicing, this was found to be the case. Large amounts of humanized mouse antibody produced by splicing could be injected into human beings without adverse reactions. Humanized antibodies have been used to treat several illnesses. Recently, the principle has been applied to the therapy of allergic asthma. Mice were immunized with human IgE, producing a mouse antibody against human IgE. Several different mouse species were immunized, and the species producing an antibody against the portion of IgE that binds to the receptor on mast cells was chosen. A hybridoma was constructed from mouse plasma cells producing antibody to IgE fused with plasma cells from a mouse with multiple myeloma. The hybridoma thus produced monoclonal antibodies directed against the portion of human IgE that binds to the mast cell. Then a humanized version of this antibody was created by cleaving the small portion of the mouse antibody binding to human IgE and attaching it to the framework of a human antibody molecule.

This humanized monoclonal antibody against IgE was tested outside of the human body and found to be capable of preventing the binding of IgE to the mast cell as well as decreasing the production of IgE by human plasma cells grown in culture.

After safety testing in humans, the antibody was administered to allergic asthmatics. Results were very promising. Several beneficial effects have been achieved, including a fall in IgE levels, a decrease in IgE receptor levels on cells, a reduction of IgE mediated degranulation of cells after exposure to allergen, a decrease in the fall in pulmonary function associated with the early phase allergic response, and a similar decrease in the late phase response. Perhaps most important, administration of this antibody resulted in a decrease in symptoms and corticosteroid use. All of this was achieved without significant side effects.

In addition to the role monoclonal antibodies have in the therapy of those already afflicted with asthma, such antibodies may also play a part in prevention of this condition. When studied in mice, monoclonal anti-IgE antibodies were capable of preventing initial allergic sensitization.

Monoclonal antibodies have also been employed in other arenas of the asthmatic response. For example, they have been used to block the influx of eosinophils into the lung. Eosinophils traveling from the bloodstream into the lung require attachment to a "docking port" on the inner surface blood vessel wall. This attachment stops their flow through the bloodstream and allows them to leave the bloodstream and gain access to the bronchi. There appear to be two very important docking ports (known as adhesion molecules) employed by the eosinophil for this purpose. One of these is known as ICAM1 and the other as VLA4; the latter may be of particular importance because it is used only by the eosinophil and the lymphocyte. Armed with this knowledge, investigators have constructed a monoclonal antibody to VLA4 and administered it to "allergic-asthmatic" sheep. The antibody not only prevented eosinophil influx into the lung but also attenuated the late phase allergic reaction and blocked the increase in bronchial hyperresponsiveness normally associated with that reaction.

As discussed earlier, interleukin 5 is a cytokine that is responsible for eosinophil production and the prolongation of the life of the eosinophil. It plays an important role in eosinophil activation and migration during the allergic-asthmatic response. A monoclonal antibody against IL-5 has been shown in a mouse model of asthma to reduce the number of eosinophils migrating to the lung and to decrease damage to the lung that normally occurs with this migration.

Thus humanized monoclonal antibodies to IgE have been administered to humans and found to be effective in the therapy of asthma, and monoclonal antibodies against VLA4 and IL-5 have been evaluated in animals and have been shown to reduce asthmatic inflammation.

## Improvements in Immunotherapy

As we saw in chapter 5, immunotherapy is the administration of allergens to sensitive individuals in gradually increasing doses over a prolonged period of time. As presently performed, the process is intended to produce a decreased sensitivity to the allergen, therefore preventing asthma when the substance is inhaled.

In its broadest sense however, immunotherapy refers to any form of administration of an immunogen (antigen) in order to favorably manipulate the immune response. New forms of immunotherapy for allergic asthma presently being evaluated have the potential of totally eliminating allergy by producing tolerance. These forms include *gene vaccination*, *peptide immunotherapy*, and *recombinant DNA modified allergen administration*.

### Gene vaccination

In gene vaccination, a gene encoding for the production of the allergen is injected into the allergic patient. This gene is administered via a plasmid. Plasmids are circular, independently self-replicating, bacterial genes (fig. 7.1). Recombinant plasmids can be constructed through molecular biology techniques. These recombinant plasmids retain their ability to self-replicate and, by virtue of the ligation of the desired gene into the plasmid, manufacture the product of the ligated gene segment. Thus, for example, the ragweed gene for the production of ragweed allergen can be ligated into a plasmid. The plasmid then will produce the allergen. The injection of plasmid encoded ragweed allergen gene into an animal results in the synthesis, within the animal, of the product of the gene (ragweed allergen). The animal will "self-produce" the allergen, as the plasmid has been incorporated into its own tissue.

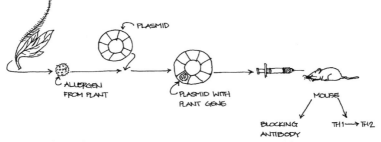

FIG. 7.1. Plasmids are circular, self-replicating bacterial genes. They can be combined, through the use of DNA recombinant technology, with a gene from a plant that produces an allergen. The injection of this recombinant plasmid into an animal results in a perpetual "immunization" and a shift from a TH2 to a TH1 lymphocyte profile.

Experiments using plasmid ligated allergen genes which produce large amounts of allergen within an animal have been shown to cause a shift from the TH2 to the TH1 profile with the production of interferon gamma (which down-regulates allergy) and blocking antibody (see chapter 5). What's more, this can be done without the production of an allergic reaction, thus eliminating one of the disadvantages of allergen immunotherapy as it is presently performed. So immunization with plasmid DNA encoding allergen antigens potentially can produce a perpetual "immunization" to allergen and "down regulation" of the allergic response.

The other fascinating aspect of this research is that through it we have learned that the bacterial structure of the plasmid favors the development of THI (versus TH2) immune profiles. It has been hypothesized that the increase in allergy per se observed over the past 50 years is a result of modern use of vaccines and antibiotics which prevent bacterial infection (and therefore exposure to bacteria) in childhood. According to this thinking, children in modern times, because of the protection afforded against bacterial infections by vaccines and antibiotics, have a higher incidence of allergy because they do not undergo bacterial-induced immune stimulation and therefore fail to develop THI cells. The administration of this type of plasmid allergen gene encoded immunization has the additional fringe benefit of inducing a THI profile (by exposing the recipient to bacterial DNA) creating tolerance to allergen.

### Peptide immunotherapy

A radically different approach to immunotherapy is to employ what are known as *peptide epitopes* of the allergens. All allergens are complex and fairly large protein molecules. Proteins are made up of connected smaller molecules known as peptides. Only very small segments of each peptide are immunogenic. That is, only these small peptides induce an immune response when injected or an allergic response when inhaled. These small peptide segments are known as epitopes.

New technology has allowed us to define the peptide sequences of large protein allergen molecules. With the ability to sequence proteins, we have been able to isolate the peptide segments responsible for the development of the immune response.

Certain peptide epitopes, when part of the whole allergen molecule, stimulate T-cells to help the plasma cell make allergic antibody and tend to create a TH2 profile. However, the peptide epitope itself, separated from the whole molecule, produces a state of tolerance. These epitopes can be synthesized in large amounts through the use of recombinant DNA technology. Immunization of asthmatics allergic to cats with these T-cell recognized epitope peptides from cat allergen proteins results in the development of tolerance. That is, instead of developing an immune response to cat allergen, the individual receiving the peptide injections becomes tolerant to exposure and no longer reacts to inhalation of cat allergen.

Tolerance develops because small peptides bypass what are known as antigen-presenting cells. Antigen-presenting cells are the cells that capture antigen (allergen) and present the antigen in a processed form to the T-cell. In order for an immune response to occur they must be involved in this preliminary processing and presentation arrangement. The small peptides escape being processed by the antigen-presenting cell and go directly to the T-cell. This direct exposure induces tolerance (fig. 7.2).

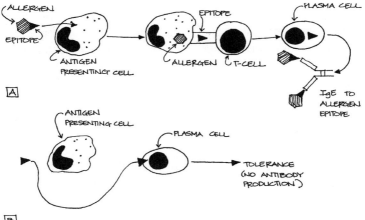

FIG. 7.2. Large proteins are processed by antigen-presenting cells and presented to T-cells (panel A), which then induce antibody formation by plasma cells. In contrast, the isolated peptide epitope induces tolerance, because it bypasses the antigen-presenting cell (panel B).

### Recombinant allergen fragments

Large recombinant allergen fragments can be constructed that are the right size to produce blocking antibody but the wrong size to unite with IgE on mast cells. Because they do not have the potential therefore to produce an adverse response during the immunization process, allergen immunotherapy can be accomplished much more quickly since larger doses can be given over a shorter period of time.

## Other Experimental Approaches

A number of other experimental approaches show promise. Although not in the same stage of development as, for example, monoclonal antibody therapy, they have significant potential from a theoretical standpoint.

### Soluble IL-4 receptors

As you will recall, IL-4 is the cytokine responsible for the production of IgE antibody. IL-4 acts on cells by combining with a receptor at the surface of those cells. This combination sends signals to the nucleus of the cell that encode for the production of IgE. The receptor for IL-4 has been isolated and can be produced in large amounts through recombinant DNA technology. Theoretically this receptor, in a soluble form, could be injected into the body and combine with IL-4 before the IL-4 reached the cell surface receptor. This type of competitive inhibition is a technique that has been employed in many other forms of therapy.

### Interferon gamma therapy

As mentioned, interferon gamma down-regulates the TH2 cell response. It interferes with IL-4 induced IgE synthesis. Thus, theoretically, altered forms of interferon gamma (which have no toxicity) could be constructed and administered to reduce IgE synthesis.

### Interference with viral adhesion

In order for viruses to enter the respiratory tract, they must combine with "docking ports" much like those required for eosinophils to enter the lung. For example, the docking port for the rhinovirus, the most common cause of colds, is known as ICAM1. Blocking ICAM1 prevents the rhinovirus from attaching to the nasal lining. Thus molecules designed to prevent the adhesion of rhinovirus to ICAM1 potentially would be capable of preventing asthma that is due to respiratory tract infections. A compound known as WIN, which fits over the cap of the virus, is being studied.

So the future for asthma sufferers is promising. Great leaps are being made as techniques derived from sister sciences such as molecular biology are applied to the field of allergy and immunology. If we see as much progress over the next three decades as we have in the last three, we can anticipate a much greater degree of control than exists today, and we may even be able to eliminate some forms of the condition.

# Appendix

Much information is available to the asthmatic. Specific self-help programs, which can be obtained from a number of sources, complement the information found in *Understanding Asthma*. The organizations listed here can help asthmatics understand the disease and learn how to manage it.

American Academy of Allergy, Asthma, and Immunology
611 East Wells Street
Milwaukee, Wisconsin 53202
(800) 822-ASTHMA (800) 822–2762

American College of Allergy, Asthma, and Immunology
85 West Algonquin Road
Arlington Heights, Illinois 60005
(800) 842–7777

These two organizations consist of physicians dedicated to the care of the asthmatic patient. Their goals are to foster education and research in allergy and asthma and to assist those affected. Educational publications,videotapes, and a list of board-certified allergists-immunologists can be obtained through both organizations.

National Jewish Medical and Research Center
1400 Jackson Street
Denver, Colorado 80206
(800) 423–8891

The physician staff at the National Jewish Medical and Research Center is actively engaged in the care of the asthmatic patient as well as in doing research regarding the causes of this illness. The center can supply educational material and a list of qualified physicians in a patient's geographical area.

The National Institutes of Health (NIH) supports an extensive range of research programs as well as patient education projects coordinated through the National Heart, Lung, and Blood Institute (NHLBI) and the National Institute of Allergy and Infectious Disease (NIAID). NIH estimates that it spent $92 million on asthma research in 1997 and $99 million in 1998, with $107 million being proposed for 1999.

The areas of research include genetics of asthma, pathogenesis and mechanisms of asthma, epidemiological research, clinical studies, environmental intervention in the primary prevention of asthma in children, Center for Disease Control and Prevention Program, and research translation: dissemination and education.

Probably the most important aspect of this activity is the National Asthma Education and Prevention Program (NAEPP), which is under the direction of the National Heart, Lung, and Blood Institute. This program has a great deal of information to offer the public and is responsible for the production of *Guidelines for the Diagnosis and Management of Asthma*, frequently mentioned in this text. Their information center provides educational material for patients that will complement the guidelines, which were intended for physicians. They also offer an asthma self-management program entitled "Breathe Easier," which is designed to assist adult asthmatics in the management of their disease. They can be reached at:

National Asthma Education and Prevention Program
National Heart, Lung, and Blood Institute
Information Center
P.O. Box 30105
Bethesda, Maryland 20854–0105
(301) 251–1222 (Information regarding other programs at NIH can also be obtained from this number.)

Asthma and Allergy Foundation of America
1125 15th Street, N.W., Suite 502
Washington, D.C. 20005
(800) 7-ASTHMA (800) 727–8462

The Asthma and Allergy Foundation of America has one specific goal—to assist patients with allergy and asthma. Self-management programs provided include "Asthma Care Training for Kids" ("A.C.T."), which is intended for children 7–12 years of age and "You Can Control Asthma," designed for children 8–12 years of age. The foundation offers educational material and has local support groups in many areas.

Allergy and Asthma Network/Mothers of Asthmatics, Inc.
3554 Chain Bridge Road, Suite 200
Fairfax, Virginia 22030–2709
(800) 878–4403

This organization, formed by the mother of an asthmatic child, was originally known as Mothers of Asthmatics. It offers educational material for asthmatics.

American Lung Association
(800) LUNG-USA (800) 586–4872

The American Lung Association offers a self-management program entitled "Open Airways at School" intended for children 8–11 years of age. It also supplies educational materials and has local support groups in many areas.

National Technical Information Service
5285 Port Royal Road
Springfield, Virginia 22161
(703) 487–4650

This organization offers several self-management programs for children, including "Air Power" (9–13), "Air Wise" (8–13),

"Living with Asthma" (8–13), and "Open Airways" (4–12). The service also offers educational material.

All of these organizations offer superb self-help guides in the form of written material and audio/visual aids such as videotapes. The asthmatic can receive information on how to properly use a metered dose inhaler, how to take peak flow measurements, how to avoid allergen exposure, and how to deal with exercise asthma, among other topics. The information is generally easy to understand and of great practical value. Much of it is supplied without charge. As noted, two of these organizations, the American Lung Association and the Asthma and Allergy Foundation of America, have local support groups, which hold meetings and offer other services to the asthmatic. Many of the organizations also have Web sites; addresses are listed below.

Allergy Internet Resources—http://www.immune.com/allergy/allabc.html
This Web site is a link to other Web sites with information about allergies and asthma.

The American Lung Association—http://www.lungusa.org
The American Lung Association, which is affiliated with the American Thoracic Society, offers information not only about asthma but about other lung diseases as well.

The American Thoracic Society—http://www.thoracic.org
The American Thoracic Society offers interesting items such as "News and Updates," "Local Chapters," and "Assemblies and Committees."

The Asthma and Allergy Foundation of America—http://www.aafa.org

This foundation publishes a newsletter, *Advance*, which can be found on the Web site and which provides a great deal of information regarding childhood asthma.

Asthma Online—http://www.asthma-online.com
This Web site helps patients become better informed. It contains numerous highlights, including "Frequently Asked Questions."

The Global Initiative for Asthma Campaign—http://www. ginasthma.com
The Global Initiative for Asthma Campaign is a project by the National Heart, Lung, and Blood Institute, the National Institutes of Health, and the World Health Organization. This organization has also published a set of guidelines known as the *GINA (Global Initiative for Asthma) Guidelines.*

JAMA Asthma Information Center—http://www.ama-assn.org/asthma
The JAMA Asthma Information Center Web site is produced by the *Journal of the American Medical Association.*

The National Asthma Campaign—http://www.asthma.org.uk
This site, based in the United Kingdom, offers a Junior Asthma Club through which children can learn about their disease.

National Jewish Medical and Research Center—http://www. national-jewish.org
This Web site, for patients and health care providers, offers more than 285 pages of information as well as addresses of other respiratory associations.

# Glossary

**Allergen** A substance that produces the allergic response, usually organic (alive or once alive) and harmless to most individuals. Examples of allergens known to cause asthma are pollens, dust mites, and animal danders.

**Allergy** An aberrant immune response, or abnormal reactivity to normally harmless substances.

**Alveoli** Air sacs at the end of the bronchioles that expand as we inhale, thus providing oxygen for the circulating blood.

**Antibody** Proteins produced by our body that help defend against infection by combining with and killing or immobilizing infectious invaders such as bacteria.

**Anticholinergic agents** Drugs used to relax the smooth muscle of the lung, which they do by blocking reflex bronchospasm.

**Antileukotriene drugs** Agents that prevent the activity of leukotrienes (chemicals that cause contraction of the smooth muscle in the lung and produce inflammation).

**Atopy** A group of inherited diseases caused by allergy and including allergic asthma, allergic rhinitis, and atopic dermatitis.

**Beta-adrenergic agents** Agents that relax the smooth muscle of the lung and thus increase the airways. They are the most potent bronchodilator (smooth muscle relaxants).

**Bronchi and bronchioles** The tubes (bronchi being the larger) that carry air from the trachea to the bottom of the lung.

**Bronchial hyperresponsiveness** An exaggerated response of the bronchi and bronchioles to stimuli known to cause asthma. It is a hallmark of the condition.

**Bronchial tree** Bronchus and bronchioles. The term refers to their resemblance to a tree, the bronchus being the trunk and the bronchioles being the branches.

**Broncho-constrictive reflex** The reflex produced by irritation of the nerve endings of the lung resulting in contraction of the smooth muscle of the lung.

**Bronchodilatation** Relaxation of the smooth muscle of the bronchi, which increases the diameter of the airways.

**Cationic protein** A substance contained in eosinophils that is highly toxic to the lining of the bronchial tubes.

**Chemokines** Chemicals released by cells. They are chemotactic and cause cells to come to an area of the body.

**Chemotactic factors** Factors that call forth cells to an area of the body. They are released during the allergic reaction and call cells to the lungs.

**Corticosteroid** An anti-inflammatory drug that, through many actions, reduces the inflammation producing asthma. These are the most potent drugs for treating the condition.

**Cromolyn sodium** A long-term controller drug thought to have disease modifying activity in the treatment of asthma.

**Cyclic AMP** A chemical that can relax the smooth muscle of the bronchi, thus serving as the target for certain drugs. For example, beta-adrenergic agents increase cyclic AMP production.

**Cytokines** Chemicals produced by cells that cause changes in other cells. There is a cytokine pattern for allergic disease. The cytokines of allergic disease are made by TH2 cells and consist of IL-4, IL-5, IL-10, and IL-13.

**Degranulation** The process by which a cell releases its internal contents into the tissues.

**Disease modifying agents** Drugs that actually affect the inflammation of asthma, therefore perhaps modifying the course of the disease and possibly preventing lung damage. These drugs are usually beneficial over the long term rather than immediately.

**Dust mite** An organism that is the major allergen in house dust.

**Edema** Swelling, a component of inflammation. In asthma it is due to leakage of serum from blood vessels and is one of the causes of narrowing of the airways.

**Elastase** An enzyme made by neutrophils and other cells. It destroys elastic tissue, which helps hold the bronchi open, and thus can reduce resistance to forces that cause narrowing of the airways.

**Elastic tissue** Tissue in the lung that helps keep the bronchioles open.

**Environmental control** The avoidance of allergens and other substances known to trigger asthma.

**Eosinophil** A cell that is operative in the production of asthma. It is called to the lung during an asthmatic episode, and its contents can be damaging to the bronchi.

**Epithelial cells** Cells that line the surfaces of organs (skin is composed of epithelial cells). In the respiratory tract, epithelial cells line the surfaces of the bronchi.

**Extrinsic asthma** Asthma produced by allergies (allergic asthma).

**Fibroblast** Cells that produce ground substance. These cells are thought to participate in the scarring or fibrosis process that can occur in the lung, since ground substance production is a component of this scarring.

**Fibrosis** Scarring that occurs as a result of damage to tissue.

**Gastroesophageal reflux** The reflux of stomach contents into the swallowing tube (esophagus), which can aggravate asthma.

**Ground substance** The "mortar and cement" of the lung tissue, holding the tissue together and also serving as "highways" for cell traffic.

**Histamine** One of the chemicals contained in mast cells and basophils. Histamine causes constriction of the muscle of the lung, leakage of serum from the blood vessels, and dilation of the blood vessels.

**Hybridoma** A cell produced by the fusion of two other cells and incorporating features of both "parents." Hybridomas are used to manufacture monoclonal antibodies.

**Hypertrophy** Overgrowth. Hypertrophy can occur in the muscles lining the bronchi and in asthma serves to narrow the airway.

**IgE** The antibody responsible for allergic reactions.

**Immediate allergic response** One of the two allergic responses that occur during an allergy reaction mediated by IgE antibody. The immediate response happens within 15 to 30 minutes.

**Immunoglobulin** A protein molecule that acts as an antibody, defending against certain forms of infection. There are five classes of immunoglobulins (immunoglobulin G, immunoglobulin A, immunoglobulin M, immunoglobulin D, and immunoglobulin E).

**Immunotherapy** The administration of allergy injections to help control allergic asthma. Allergens are administered in gradually increasing doses over a long period of time to reduce the patient's sensitivity to them.

**Inflammation** A process characterized by heat, redness, and swelling, typically resulting from an influx of cells into a particular area of the body. Usually called forth to fight foreign invaders, the cells produce what is known as the inflammatory response, causing damage not only to the invader but also to the surrounding tissue.

**Interleukin-4 (IL-4)** A cytokine produced by TH2 cells that enhances the production of the antibody for allergy, IgE.

**Interleukin-5 (IL-5)** A cytokine produced by TH2 cells that enhances the life span and activates eosinophils, one of the major effector cells of asthma.

**Interleukin-10 (IL-10)** A cytokine produced by TH2 cells that enhances the allergic response and dampens the activity of TH1 cells.

**Interleukin-13 (IL-13)** A cytokine that assists IL-4 in the production of the antibody for allergy, IgE. It is made by TH2 cells.

**Intracellular organisms** Organisms that invade the body and live within cells. A classic example is the tuberculosis organism.

**Intrinsic asthma** Asthma not related to allergy. Symptoms are similar to those produced in allergic asthma, but the sufferer has no allergies. The illness is due to other precipitants, including infections, respiratory irritants, and weather conditions.

**Kallikreins** Chemicals produced by mast cells that can participate in inflammation characteristic of asthma. They can irritate the nerve supply to the lung and produce what is known as reflex bronchospasm.

**Late phase response** One of the two allergic responses that occur during an allergy reaction mediated by IgE antibody. The late phase response happens 4 to 6 hours later.

**Leukotrienes** Chemicals contained within mast cells, basophils, eosinophils, and monocytes. They cause many of the manifestations of asthma, including contraction of smooth muscle, increased bronchial hyperresponsiveness, activation of eosinophils, and activation of fibroblasts.

**Lymphocytes** Cells that participate in the production of asthma. Lymphocytes are divided into two types. The B-lymphocyte produces antibody and is thus responsible for the production of the allergic antibody, IgE. The T-lymphocyte is the orchestrator of the immune response and is divided into a TH1 and TH2 population. The TH1 cell defends us against intracellular organisms such as tuberculosis. The TH2 cell enhances the production of allergic antibody and is overactive in allergic asthma.

**Macrophage** A cell active in asthma. These cells normally fight infections, and their contents can be damaging to the lung.

**Major basic protein** A substance contained in eosinophils that is highly toxic to the lining of the bronchial tubes.

**Mast cell** A cell containing histamine and other chemicals that produce asthma. The mast cell releases these chemicals in the lung, thus causing many of the condition's symptoms.

**Metered dose inhaler** A device used to deliver aerosolized drugs. It administers a standard (metered) dose with each actuation.

**Methacholine** A chemical used to test for bronchial hyperresponsiveness. When inhaled it causes constriction of the smooth muscle of the lung and therefore narrows the airway. Asthmatics are far more sensitive to methacholine than are people without the condition.

**Methacholine challenge test** Used to diagnose asthma in some patients. Asthmatics are overly sensitive to methacholine, responding in an exaggerated fashion to the inhalation of this drug; the response is characterized by constriction of the smooth muscle of the bronchi.

**Monoclonal antibodies** Antibodies produced in a hybridoma, which is a cell formed from the fusion of two separate cell lines. One of the cell lines is capable of manufacturing antibodies in large amounts and the other of growing in cell culture indefinitely. When these two cell lines are fused, large amounts of (monoclonal) antibodies directed against a particular substance can be produced.

**Nedocromil** A long-term controller drug thought to have disease modifying activity in the treatment of asthma.

**Neural endopeptidases** Chemicals that destroy neuropeptides.

**Neuropeptides**: Substances released from nerve endings that can make asthma worse by contracting the smooth muscle of the lungs and increasing the permeability of the blood vessels. Neuropeptides are released when the lining of the lung is irritated or during the allergic response.

**Neutrophils** Cells that fight infection by ingesting germs and other invaders. They can be overactive in certain cases of asthma but are not normally characteristic of this illness.

**Peak flow** The fastest rate of air flow through the bronchus. Peak flow measurements can be performed at home with a portable peak flow meter.

**Peptide immunotherapy** Peptides are small sections of very large protein molecules and can be used in immunization to produce tolerance to the large protein from which they were separated.

**Plasma cells** Cells that manufacture antibodies.

**Plasmid** A circular, independently self-replicating bacterial gene. Plasmids can be used as vectors of genes. That is, genes can be inserted into a plasmid and the plasmid will then produce the gene product as long as it is alive and replicating. Injection of the plasmid into an individual will result in the production of the gene product for many years, which can immunize the injected individual against the substance. In the future, plasmids may be used to immunize against allergen gene products.

**Platelet activating factor** A chemical produced by mast cells that can cause constriction of the smooth muscle of the bronchi.

**Prostaglandins** Chemicals produced by mast cells, some of which can constrict smooth muscle and enhance permeability of blood vessels.

**Pulmonary function test** A test that measures breathing ability, especially useful in asthma since it measures the rate of air flow through the bronchi.

**Reflex bronchospasm** A reflex that is not under conscious control and is mediated by what is known as the autonomic nervous system. It occurs when nerve endings in the bronchi are irritated. This irritation sends a message to the brain, which returns a message to the bronchial muscle producing contraction and narrowing the airway.

**Rhinitis** Inflammation of the nose, which produces sneezing, runny nose, nasal congestion, and postnasal drainage.

**Sinusitis** Inflammation of the sinus cavities surrounding the nose and connected to it by tubes. Sinusitis can aggravate asthma.

**Skin test** Used to determine the presence of allergy. The test involves placing an allergen on the skin and puncturing the site or injecting the allergen into the skin.

**Spacer devices** Devices that are connected to metered dose inhalers to facilitate the inhalation of aerosols.

**Symptom treaters** Drugs that control the symptoms of asthma but do not alter the course of the disease or prevent long-term damage. They are also known as "quick relief medications."

**Theophylline** A drug used to relax the smooth muscle of the bronchi and thus cause bronchodilatation.

**TH1 lymphocytes** A subset of the helper T-lymphocyte. They are operative in our defense against intracellular infections such as tuberculosis.

**TH2 lymphocytes** A subset of the population of T-helper lymphocytes. They enhance the allergic response by increasing the production of allergic antibody (IgE).

**Trachea** The large air tube connected to the pharynx that carries air into the bronchi. The trachea divides into the bronchial tubes.

**Transforming growth factor beta (TGF beta)** A chemical manufactured by many cells that can activate fibroblasts and cause them to produce ground substances. It thus may be active in causing lung scarring (fibrosis).

**Upper respiratory tract viral infection** The common cold.

# Index